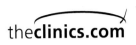

theclinics.com

# CRITICAL CARE
# NURSING CLINICS
## OF NORTH AMERICA

Nurses' Experiences in War
and Disaster: Lessons Learned
and Needs Identified

GUEST EDITORS
Catherine Wilson Cox, RN, PhD, CCRN, CEN,
CCNS, CAPT, NC, USN (RC) and
Janet Fraser Hale, PhD, APRN-BC, FNP, COL,
AN, USAR (Ret)

D1225368

CONSULTING EDITOR
Janet Foster, PhD, RN, CNS, CCRN

March 2008 • Volume 20 • Number 1

**SAUNDERS**

An Imprint of Elsevier, Inc.
PHILADELPHIA    LONDON    TORONTO    MONTREAL    SYDNEY    TOKYO

**W.B. SAUNDERS COMPANY**
*A Division of Elsevier Inc.*

Elsevier Inc., 1600 John F. Kennedy Blvd., Suite 1800, Philadelphia, PA 19103-2899.

http://www.theclinics.com

**CRITICAL CARE NURSING CLINICS OF NORTH AMERICA**
March 2008
Editor: Ali Gavenda

Volume 20, Number 1
ISSN 0899-5885
ISBN-13: 978-1-4160-6061-1
ISBN-10: 1-4160-6061-8

The ideas and opinions expressed in *Critical Care Nursing Clinics of North America* do not necessarily reflect those of the Publisher. The Publisher does not assume any responsibility for any injury and/or damage to persons or property arising out of or related to any use of the material contained in this periodical. The reader is advised to check the appropriate medical literature and the product information currently provided by the manufacturer of each drug to be administered to verify the dosage, the method and duration of administration, or contraindications. It is the responsibility of the treating physician or other health care professional, relying on independent experience and knowledge of the patient, to determine drug dosages and the best treatment for the patient. Mention of any product in this issue should not be construed as endorsement by the contributors, editors, or the Publisher of the product or manufacturers' claims.

*Critical Care Nursing Clinics of North America* (ISSN 0899-5885) is published quarterly by Elsevier Inc., 360 Park Avenue South, New York, NY 10010-1710. Months of issue are March, June, September, and December. Business and Editorial Offices: 1600 John F. Kennedy Blvd., Suite 1800, Philadelphia, PA 19103-2899. Customer Service Office: 6277 Sea Harbor Drive, Orlando, FL 32887-4800. Periodicals postage paid at New York, NY and additional mailing offices. Subscription prices are $120.00 per year for US individuals, $212.00 per year for US institutions, $63.00 per year for US students and residents, $155.00 per year for Canadian individuals, $260.00 per year for Canadian institutions, $166.00 per year for international individuals, $260.00 per year for international institutions and $86.00 per year for Canadian and foreign students/residents. To receive student/resident rate, orders must be accompanied by name of affiliated institution, data of term, and the *signature* of program/residency coordinator on institution letterhead. Orders will be billed at individual rate until proof of status is received. Foreign air speed delivery is included in all *Clinics* subscription prices. All prices are subject to change without notice. **POSTMASTER:** Send address changes to *Critical Care Nursing Clinics of North America*, Elsevier Periodicals Customer Service, 6277 Sea Harbor Drive, Orlando, FL 32887-4800. **Customer Service: 1-800-654-2452 (US). From outside of the US, call 1-407-345-4000.**

*Critical Care Nursing Clinics of North America* is covered in *International Nursing Index, Nursing Citation Index, Cumulative Index to Nursing and Allied Health Literature, and RNdex Top 100*.

Printed in the United States of America.

# CONSULTING EDITOR

**JANET FOSTER, PhD, RN, CNS, CCRN,** Assistant Professor, Texas Woman's University, College of Nursing, Houston, Texas

# GUEST EDITORS

**CATHERINE WILSON COX, RN, PhD, CCRN, CEN, CCNS, CAPT, NC, USN (RC),** Assistant Professor, School of Nursing & Health Studies, Georgetown University, Washington, District of Columbia

**JANET FRASER HALE, PhD, APRN-BC, FNP, COL, AN, USAR (Ret),** Associate Dean and Professor; and Director of Interdisciplinary and Community Partnerships, Graduate School of Nursing, University of Massachusetts, Worcester, Massachusetts

# CONTRIBUTORS

**LORETTA J. AIKEN, RN, MSN,** Clinical Nurse Specialist, Cardiology and Cardiothoracic Surgery, National Naval Medical Center, Bethesda, Maryland

**PATRICE BIBEAU, RN, MSN, CCRN, CDR, NC, USN,** Associate Director, Cardiovascular and Critical Care Services, National Naval Medical Center, Bethesda, Maryland

**ELIZABETH J. BRIDGES, PhD, RN, CCNS, Lt Col, USAFR, NC,** Individual Mobilization Augmentee — Director, Clinical Investigations Facility, 60th Medical Group, Travis AFB, California; Assistant Professor, Biobehavioral Nursing and Health Systems, University of Washington School of Nursing; and Clinical Nurse Researcher, University of Washington Medical Center, Seattle, Washington

**BARBIE CILENTO, RN, M Ed, MSN,** Clinical Nurse Specialist, Critical Care Department, National Naval Medical Center, Bethesda, Maryland

**SEAN T. COLLINS, PhD(c), MS, APRN-BC, Lt Col, MA ANG, NC,** Graduate School of Nursing, University of Massachusetts Worcester; and Medical Group Commander, 104th FW, Barnes Air National Guard Base, Westfield, Massachusetts

**CATHERINE WILSON COX, RN, PhD, CCRN, CEN, CCNS, CAPT, NC, USN (RC),** Assistant Professor, School of Nursing & Health Studies, Georgetown University, Washington, District of Columbia

**JANET FABLING, RD, CNSD, CSP,** Chief, Medical Nutrition Therapy, Madigan Army Medical Center, Tacoma, Washington

**MARY E. FREYLING, RN, MS, CCRN, CCNS, LTC, AN, USA,** Clinical Nurse Specialist, Tripler Army Medical Center, Surgical Product Line, Honolulu, Hawaii

**JANET FRASER HALE, PhD, APRN-BC, FNP, COL, AN, USAR (Ret),** Associate Dean and Professor; and Director of Interdisciplinary and Community Partnerships, Graduate School of Nursing, University of Massachusetts, Worcester, Massachusetts

**JANIE HEATH, PhD, APRN-BC, ANP, ACNP,** Associate Dean, Academic Nursing Practice, Medical College of Georgia School of Nursing, Augusta, Georgia

**MARY S. HULL, RN, MSN, APN, LTC, AN, USA,** Nurse Manager/Officer in Charge, Inpatient Psychiatry, Landstuhl Regional Medical Center, Landstuhl, Germany

**PATRICIA WATTS KELLEY, PhD, RN, FNP, GNP, CAPT, NC, USN,** Assistant Professor, TriService Nursing Research Program, Uniformed Services University of the Health Sciences, Bethesda, Maryland

**DEBORAH J. KENNY, RN, PhD, LTC, AN, USA,** Executive Director, TriService Nursing Research Program, Uniformed Services University of the Health Sciences, Bethesda, Maryland

**KAREN S. KESTEN, RN, MSN, CCRN, PCCN, CCNS,** Assistant Professor, Georgetown University School of Nursing & Health Studies, Washington, District of Columbia

**ANN KOBIELA KETZ, MN, RN, AOCNS, CPT, AN, USA,** Department of Emergency Medicine, Landstuhl Regional Medical Center, Landstuhl; and 212th Combat Support Hospital, Miesau, Germany

**SANDRA L. LEIBY, RN, MSN, APRN-BC,** Instructor, Graduate School of Nursing, University of Massachusetts, Worcester, Massachusetts

**MARGUERITE T. LITTLETON-KEARNEY, PhD, RN, FAAN,** Associate Professor of Nursing, Department of Acute and Chronic Care, Johns Hopkins School of Nursing; and Associate Professor of Medicine, Department of Anesthesia/Critical Care Medicine, Johns Hopkins School of Medicine, Baltimore, Maryland

**EDDIE LOPEZ, RN, MSN, LCDR, NC, USN,** Department Head, Critical Care Department, National Naval Medical Center, Bethesda, Maryland

**ROBERT MARTINDALE, MD, PhD,** Professor of Surgery and Director of Medical Nutrition Services, Oregon Health and Science University, Portland, Oregon

**MARY S. MCCARTHY, PhD, RN, CNSN,** Clinical Nurse Researcher, Nursing Research Service, Madigan Army Medical Center, Tacoma, Washington

**STEPHANIE ANN MEYER, MS, RD, MAJ, SP, USA,** Chief, Medical Nutrition Therapy, Landstuhl Regional Medical Center, Landstuhl, Germany

**KIMBERLY J. NEWELL, RN, MSN, CCRN, CNS, CDR, NC, USN,** Head, Education and Training Department, Naval Hospital Camp Pendleton, Camp Pendleton, California

**TIMOTHY PEARMAN, PhD,** Clinical Associate Professor of Psychiatry & Neurology; and Director, Patricia Trost-Friedler Center for Psychosocial Oncology, Tulane University Medical Center, New Orleans, Louisiana

**JACQUELINE RHOADS, PhD, APRN, ACNP-BC, ANP-C, CCRN, FAANP,** Professor, Director Primary Care Community Health Public Health Nursing Program, LSUHSC School of Nursing, New Orleans, Louisiana

**SUSAN RICK, DNS, APRN,** Associate Professor, Mental Health Nursing, LSUHSC School of Nursing, New Orleans, Louisiana

**JOSEPH SCHMELZ, PhD, RN, Lt Col, USAF, NC (Ret),** Director, Institutional Review Board and Associate Professor/Research, School of Nursing, University of Texas Health Science Center at San Antonio (UTHSCSA), San Antonio, Texas

**LYNN A. SLEPSKI, MSN, RN, CCNS, USPHS,** Senior Public Health Advisor, U.S. Public Health Service, Risk Management Analysis Department of Homeland Security, Washington, District of Columbia

**JOHN J. WHITCOMB, PhD, RN, CCRN, CDR, NC, USN,** Nurse Scientist, Naval Medical Center Portsmouth, Portsmouth, Virginia

CONTRIBUTORS

# CONTENTS

Early in the author's deployment in the United States Air Force to southern Iraq, his unit was exposed to the first of many mass casualties sent to his Expeditionary Medical Support System unit. Within minutes of the injured military members' arrival, the four-bed evaluation station was transformed into an open bay trauma room where patients were treated and supported until they could be evacuated to more definitive care. Patients were transitioned with awe-inspiring speed and professionalism to Critical Care Air Transport teams for care during aeromedical evacuation. The lessons learned from the frequency of these events are valuable to any similar transport case with critically ill and injured patients.

Based in Kuwait 3 years apart, the authors recount how nurses and corps staff, along with their physician counterparts, came together to form well-run medical facilities under adverse circumstances. Their respective hospitals became competent organizations because of specific formulas for success, along with preparation, identification of required skill sets, and making improvements based on experience. This article describes the training of medical, nursing, and corps staff, the facilities and resources required for managing casualties, and some of the more commonly encountered combat injuries and conditions.

The Synergy Model for Patient Care, developed by the American Association of Critical-Care Nurses (AACN), demonstrates that positive patient outcomes are achieved when patient characteristics are matched with nurse competencies. Through the vivid realities in the daily journal of a military ICU nurse taking care of patients in Iraq, a virtual triad learning experience provided academic, clinical, and personal support. This article describes how effective nursing practice, whether providing direct patient care in the United States or in a military ICU in Iraq, must be centered around the needs and characteristics of patients. Acute and critically ill patients in a military ICU in Iraq have unique needs and require nurses with competent skills to help promote optimal outcomes.

This article has been written by four staff members from the Critical Care Department at the National Naval Medical Center in Bethesda, Maryland. They are part of a large and extremely sophisticated medical response team who cares for the injured when they return to the United States. This article covers the interdisciplinary teamwork that is vital to the care of catastrophic war injuries and shows how detailed treatment plans are formulated for each casualty. It describes the unique and profound emotional responses of the staff members who are instrumental in the recuperation of the service member. It also tells of the joy of recovery from horrific injuries, and the intense dedication of staff members to the military wounded.

Nursing in a critical care environment is stressful, particularly when patients are young, previously healthy soldiers who have experienced multiple severe, life-threatening injuries. These injuries not only devastate the injured soldiers and their families, but also significantly impact the nurses caring for these patients. This article discusses some stressors identified by critical care nurses in two military medical treatment facilities where the most severely injured soldiers undergo definitive care, and examines the evolution of the concept of compassion fatigue, its symptoms, and methods of coping. Examples of how the nurses currently working with these young soldiers manage their own stressors are discussed and suggestions for successful coping strategies are provided.

Traumatic amputees may experience a variety of acute and chronic pain issues, including phantom limb pain and residual limb pain. Research continues to determine the causes of these problems and to find the most appropriate and effective treatments for each of these phenomena. It is important for health care providers to be knowledgeable about the variety of treatments available, including medications, surgical procedures, complementary and alternative therapies, and self-treatment methods to ensure that amputees receive the best practices for individualized, effective pain management that they deserve.

Major trauma induces metabolic alterations that contribute to the systemic immune suppression in severely injured patients and increase the risk of infection and posttraumatic organ failure. Nutrition modulation of cellular processes has evolved into a high-priority therapy, backed by substantial scientific evidence. The appropriate selection, timing, and dose of nutrients required for metabolic resuscitation must be individualized and goal directed. Ideally, the nutritional interventions for warfighters will be developed strategically based on the extent of injuries and underlying deficiencies and will be designed to provide the nutrients necessary to balance hypermetabolic processes, heal wounds, and promote optimal recovery.

## Memories of Three Wars: A Nurse's Story
Loretta J. Aiken

This is the personal story of a civilian critical care nurse who has worked for several decades with war casualties. It begins with her memories of the Vietnam era and her reflections on that war. It then describes how the National Naval Medical Center in Bethesda, Maryland, prepared for the Desert Storm War and continues through the current war in Iraq. The article provides a glimpse of a long and meaningful nursing career and expresses the joy and satisfaction of caring for the wounded warriors of today's conflict.

## PTSD: Therapeutic Interventions Post-Katrina
Jacqueline Rhoads, Timothy Pearman, and Susan Rick

August 29, 2006, brought the largest, most deadly hurricane ever to strike the Gulf Coast. According to reports, the storm killed more than 2000 people and destroyed billions of dollars of property, with winds clocked at 160 to 175 mph. More than a million residents were displaced, many requiring care for chronic conditions who suddenly also needed care for acute stress symptoms. Today, many individuals still struggle to cope with major psychiatric posttraumatic stress disorders (PTSD). Using a case study approach, this article discusses PTSD, including what it is, how it is manifested, how to diagnose it, patient education, and how it can be managed with therapeutic interventions. Special circumstances related to children are briefly presented.

## Caring for the Caregivers and Patients Left Behind: Experiences of a Volunteer Nurse During Hurricane Katrina
Sandra L. Leiby

As a volunteer nurse deployed to New Orleans after Hurricane Katrina, the author observed the need for honest and informative leadership, for volunteer flexibility and an "I'll-do-anything" mind-set, and for more advanced disaster training. This article describes the author's experiences and highlights how she learned those lessons. She advocates learning from the experiences of responders to recent national and international relief efforts to ensure the organizational and personal preparedness needed to deal with the complex ethical, moral, legal, and medical issues during a disaster.

## Managing a Disaster Scene and Multiple Casualties Before Help Arrives
Janet Fraser Hale

As the largest group of health care professionals in the United States and a component of almost every community, nurses may be called upon to initiate the emergency response and provide initial planning for health care until local, national, or federal assistance arrives. This article will assist nurses in anticipating, preparing for, and responding to multi-casualty, high-impact events. It concludes with a discussion of triage of multi-casualties in the face of scarce resources. It includes resources for more in-depth information on prevention, preparedness and planning, and the health system's response.

# FORTHCOMING ISSUES

# RECENT ISSUES

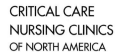

CRITICAL CARE
NURSING CLINICS
OF NORTH AMERICA

ELSEVIER
SAUNDERS

Crit Care Nurs Clin N Am 20 (2008) xi–xii

# Preface

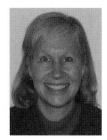 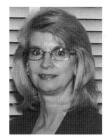

Catherine Wilson Cox,
RN, PhD, CCRN, CEN, CCNS,
CAPT, NC, USN (RC)

Janet Fraser Hale,
PhD, APRN-BC, FNP,
COL, AN, USAR (Ret)

*Guest Editors*

We are honored to coedit this special issue of *Critical Care Nursing Clinics of North America* and are proud of each author's distinctive contribution to critical care nursing practice in these unique environments. These authors have eloquently displayed their ability to translate into words the significance of their experiences and the lessons learned from the trauma of war and disaster. They also show how these lessons can be applied by their critical care nursing counterparts who work in more traditional settings with the usual populations of critical care patients. We have tried to highlight the importance of preparation and addressing postevent issues, the importance of future planning along with the value of the many lessons learned, and the development of best practices from the research along with the obvious need for much more nursing research in these arenas.

The authors range from civilian nurses working in both civilian and military facilities to those federalized for disaster response to active duty, reserve, and National Guard nurses from the Army, Air Force, and Navy. The topics covered in the articles paint a very broad picture of *Nurses' Experiences in War and Disaster: Lessons Learned and Needs Identified*. These topics range from the emotional and psychologic impact of war or disaster on patients, families, and nurses (see the articles by Collins; Freyling, Kesten, and Heath; Aiken, Bibeau, Cilento, and Lopez; Kenny and Hull; Aiken; Rhoads, Pearman, and Rick; and Leiby), the value of good collaboration, team work, and communication skills (see the articles by Collins; Whitcomb and Newell; Freyling and colleagues; Aiken and colleagues; Kenny and colleagues; Rhoads and colleagues; and Leiby), to the physiologic and pathophysiologic impact on patient needs and nursing care (see the articles by Freyling and colleagues; Aiken and colleagues; Kenny and Hull; Ketz; McCarthy, Fabling, Martindale, and Meyer; and Bridges, Schmelz, and Watts Kelley).

Approaches to direct patient care are also addressed. Evidence to support best practices is found in articles by Freyling and colleagues; Aiken and colleagues; Ketz; McCarthy and colleagues; and Bridges and colleagues. The articles by Collins; Freyling and colleagues; Rhoads and colleagues; and Leiby provide insight into the value of cultural sensitivity, reminding us that cultural norms have an impact on the care provided not only in other countries, but also within the United States. The intersection between cultural sensitivity to the Iraqi culture and applying the synergy model of the American Association of Critical Care Nurses is

0899-5885/08/$ - see front matter. Published by Elsevier Inc.
doi:10.1016/j.ccell.2007.11.001

clearly demonstrated in the article by Freyling and colleagues on caring for patients while deployed.

Educational needs are covered from all perspectives. The lessons learned from Leiby's article support the need for a minimum basic understanding of the greater picture of disaster health care anticipation and planning, regardless of the event, and the planned role for nurses, as further discussed in Fraser Hale's article. The articles by Whitcomb and Newell, Rhoads and colleagues, and Leiby on other lessons learned similarly identify the need for focused education to prepare nurses who are deploying to a war zone (Collins; Whitcomb and Newell) and in educating nurses to function as leaders in emergencies and disasters (Fraser Hale; Littleton-Kearney and Slepski). This preparation currently includes formal educational programs offering specialties, degrees, and certificates to address the unique environments and situations in which nurses are and will be needed (Littleton-Kearney and Slepski). Finally, and equally as important, are the opportunities and desperate need for research in the area of disaster nursing (Wilson Cox) and the brilliant translation of findings from military nursing research to day-to-day critical care nursing (Bridges and colleagues).

Aiken's heartfelt descriptions are extremely moving! Drawing on 40 years as a civilian nurse in veteran's and military health care facilities, she portrays unforgettable moments with the young warrior patients she cared for during three wars. She eloquently describes both the pain and rewards of nursing these very special patients, most of whom would not be patients at all had they not been physically present/working in specific environments that put them at risk for becoming patients. We appreciate all of the authors' ability to bring their experiences to life and to help the reader incorporate them for practical application in the future. Our hope is that the real-time depiction of the experiences, the vivid descriptions, and the findings presented in all the articles will contribute to readers' ability to respond and react to any high-impact event. In case of such a devastating event, we hope that readers will be able to deliver care sensitively and with the best available evidence to deal with the inevitable tragic fallout in terms of patient numbers and acuity, the heavy emotional and physical toll on nurses and their loved ones, and the communities that are involved.

We sincerely thank all the authors for bringing their experiences to life and for reminding us why we all go to work every day and of the honor we have in serving people in their moments of darkness, sadness, and greatest need. We thank the publishers for their willingness to showcase this unique aspect of nursing and to give voice to those who have had an opportunity to serve the profession in this honorable manner.

The contributions of the authors to this issue make us proud of our profession and our colleagues who have been and will be on the front lines of war and disaster nursing. May their words support and teach us, providing insights that we can apply when called upon to do so.

Catherine Wilson Cox, RN, PhD, CCRN, CEN, CCNS, CAPT, NC, USN (RC)
*School of Nursing & Health Studies*
*Gerogetown University*
*3700 Reservoir Road, NW*
*Washington, DC 20057, USA*

*E-mail address:* cwc5@georgetown.edu

Janet Fraser Hale, PhD, APRN-BC, FNP, COL, AN, USAR (Ret)
*Graduate School of Nursing*
*University of Massachusetts*
*55 Lake Avenue North*
*Worcester, MA 10655, USA*

*E-mail address:* Janet.Hale@umassmed.edu

**ELSEVIER
SAUNDERS**

Crit Care Nurs Clin N Am 20 (2008) 1–11

CRITICAL CARE
NURSING CLINICS
OF NORTH AMERICA

# Emergency Medical Support Units to Critical Care Transport Teams in Iraq

Sean T. Collins, PhD(c), MS, APRN-BC, Lt Col, MA ANG, NC[a,b,]*

[a]Graduate School of Nursing, University of Massachusetts, Worcester, MA, USA
[b]104th FW, Barnes Air National Guard Base, Westfield, MA, USA

The imagery of warfare has never been so easily accessible to the public. The sights and sounds of war can be viewed almost instantaneously on the evening news or seen on the Internet. The shadow of war has been cast upon several generations in the United States, but perhaps never with such immediate processing. Some of my earliest recollections of war were seeing clips of the Vietnam War on the daily evening news. Those news clips showed soldiers in the jungles of a distant land, carrying machine guns and helping their injured buddies. The news brought the grittiness of war into our living rooms. The carnage of war was tempered; however, the average citizen could recognize the destruction of battle.

A fascinating portrayal of the human aspects and impact of war came from one of my favorite television shows, M*A*S*H. In the series, Dr. Hawkeye Pierce, a dedicated general surgeon thrown into the chaos and destruction of the Korean War, was my hero. Hawkeye questioned why he was in an operating room (OR) so far away from home, trying to piece together the young soldiers who met their fate on the battlefield, day after day. Nonetheless, he understood that he was there to provide much-needed care and he never wavered in his professional role. The patient was always his mental anchor during the tumultuous situations he faced. The importance of having talented health care providers to save our soldiers was of great importance to him, a value that helped shape my interest in being a part of that wartime process.

## Expeditionary medical support system

In modern warfare, it is important to bring health care as close as possible to the battle, thus embracing the golden hour of trauma care. Expeditionary Medical Support System (EMEDS) is the relatively new building block of medical care provided in the combat zone [1]. Since the Korean War, sick and injured troops have been transported by helicopter from the battlefield to a location far behind the enemy lines. In these places, a Mobile Army Surgical Hospital (MASH) could provide care close to the battlefield, but at a safe distance. The Vietnam War adapted techniques used in the Korean War and perfected the "dust off," an army aeromedical evacuation (aerovac) process of bringing wounded soldiers from the battlefield to field hospitals. However, because treatment at field hospitals during the Vietnam War was limited, critically injured military members were not transported until they were stable enough to travel. The level and location of care have changed since Operation Desert Storm in Iraq, during which medical services ascertained that for care to be effective, it needed to be offered closer to the combat zone [1].

To fit within the US Air Force (USAF) Air Expeditionary model of being lean and portable, the EMEDS concept was born. The need to get to a "hot" zone quickly and efficiently forced the

The views expressed in this article are those of the author and do not reflect the official policy of the Department of the Air Force, the Department of Defense, or the US Government.

* 7R Blackberry Crescent Circle, Southwick, MA 01077.

*E-mail address:* sean.collins2@umassmed.edu

0899-5885/08/$ - see front matter. Published by Elsevier Inc.
doi:10.1016/j.ccell.2007.10.005

*ccnursing.theclinics.com*

USAF to develop a modular hospital that could flex up or shrink, based on the operational needs of a mission. It makes sense to bring only what is needed; bringing unneeded supplies and personnel is costly in time and resources. "The EMEDS concept is a phased-in deployment that develops into a theater hospital, with specialty care available in separate modular packages" [2]. Major General George Taylor, Surgeon General USAF, attributed the survival of 90% of injured combat veterans in Operation Iraqi Freedom to the EMEDS program [3].

*Concept of operations*

The basic premise of EMEDS is to create building blocks of small medical care modules that can be quickly assembled and transported to a battle site. This modular approach allows the air force great flexibility in meeting medical needs in a field of operation and reduces the footprint of medical facilities. The different EMEDS modules include the EMEDS basic, EMEDS plus 10, and the EMEDS plus 25. The EMEDS basic module consists of a two-person preventive aerospace medical team and a five-person mobile field surgical team that make up a rapid response team [4]. The surgical team, which is one of first to deploy and arrive at a designated location, travels with its required surgical equipment in backpacks. They do not have tents, so they work out of a location of opportunity, converting any building into an OR [4].

Within 24 hours, the remaining 18 members of this unit arrive, bringing with them all the tents to construct the physical EMEDS basic module. Another 12 hours later, full clinical operations can start in the module, including aerospace medicine, preventive medicine, dental care, primary care, emergency care, critical care, and surgical capability [4]. The EMEDS basic module, which has limited inpatient beds, services a deployed military force of 500 to 3000 individuals. Because this module has a limited capacity for treating ill patients for more than 24 hours, rapid aeromedical evacuation is paramount to patient care [2]. The EMEDS basic unit can perform 10 major surgeries (using one table) or 20 nonoperative trauma resuscitations in 24 hours, with supplies and equipment to provide this capability once during a 7-day period [4].

If the site of operation requires more medical assets and resources, the next echelon of EMEDS modules is activated. The EMEDS plus 10 module increases inpatient beds by 10 by adding tents and personnel to enhance care capability [4]. The last level is the EMEDS plus 25 module, which has 25 beds and more than 80 personnel, and services a deployed military force of 3000 to 5000 individuals. This module provides 24-hour care for all emergency and ambulatory medical care in an interconnected tent structure (Figs. 1 and 2). The EMEDS plus 25 provides multiple medical services, including preventive medicine, trauma resuscitation and stabilization, limited general and orthopedic surgery (using two tables)

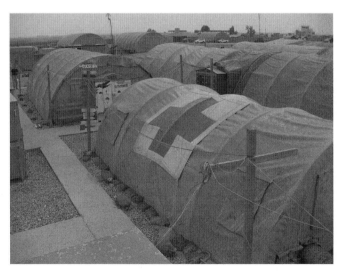

Fig. 1. Aerial view of 407th Air Expeditionary Group EMEDS.

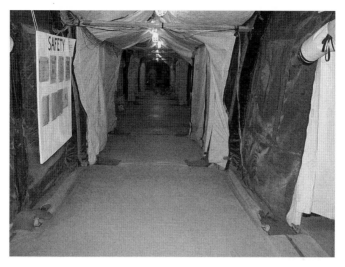

Fig. 2. Hallway of 407th Air Expeditionary Group EMEDS.

(Fig. 3), critical care, primary care, aeromedical evacuation coordination, aerospace medicine, urgent care (Figs. 4 and 5), dental care, and laboratory and radiology services [4]. The EMEDS plus 25 is a small hospital with all the resources that one would find in an American hospital.

Having been deployed to work in both an EMEDS unit and its predecessor, the Air Transportable Clinic (ATC), I can verify that the EMEDS concept of operation and layout is extremely successful. When I was deployed in 1999 during the Kosovo crisis, I set up and worked in an ATC, which arrived as tents and medical supplies on several pallets. This ATC served as the primary emergency room (ER) and sick call clinic for all deployed personnel assigned to the fighter wing, the air force equivalent of an army base. Capabilities were somewhat limited by today's military medical and nursing standards, which include advanced trauma capabilities and more medical personnel. With basic lifesaving equipment and medications in the ATC, we provided essential care to the deployed military members.

## Other roles of the Expeditionary Medical Support System plus 25

The EMEDS plus 25 offers many medical services to the base and surrounding area. At the 407th Air Expeditionary Group (AEG) EMEDS where I was stationed in Iraq, the

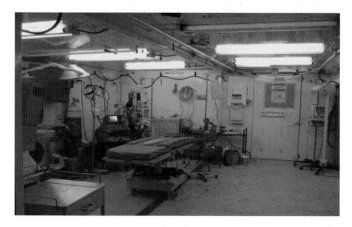

Fig. 3. Table #1 OR 407th Air Expeditionary Group EMEDS.

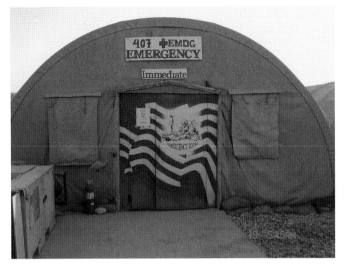

Fig. 4. 407th Air Expeditionary Group EMEDS Emergency Room door.

laboratory and pharmacy and the radiology unit were visited by many ambulatory patients. These areas were well organized and coordinated to offer a high level of service. Not only did the EMEDS provide excellent medical and nursing care but also dental care. The dental clinic was sometimes the busiest location in the facility. We had two excellent dentists, one of whom was an army dentist on an extended tour, working side by side with air force personnel. The importance of dental health is important because dental problems can impact negatively on a military mission [5].

## Aerovac and the Critical Care Air Transport team

Aerovac, whether it occurs on the battlefield, by helicopter, or by fixed-wing aircraft, certainly gets the adrenaline flowing. Not only has the military modernized its weaponry and changed the dynamics of the battlefield but it has also advanced its techniques for moving injured troops out of the combat zone. Patients are now being airlifted to more definitive care while still in critical condition. This expeditious medical evacuation ensures that injured military members receive the highest level of care as quickly as

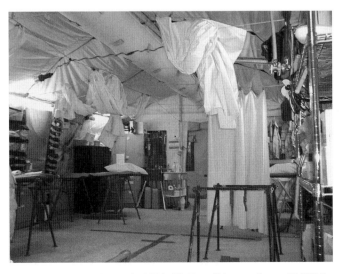

Fig. 5. Emergency Room in 407th Air Expeditionary Group EMEDS.

possible. Resources for higher levels of care can be concentrated in identified locations within the combat zone or in a regional military medical center (ie, in Europe). This regional localization of larger medical facilities allows smaller facilities to provide stabilization closer to the combat zone.

During aerovac of injured troops, critical care is provided by Critical Care Air Transport (CCAT) teams, which consist of a critical care physician, a critical care nurse, and a cardiopulmonary technician [6], with skills that may be found in the most advanced ICU in the United States. The team is responsible for monitoring and managing patients who require intensive care as they are being transferred to the appropriate level of medical care [7]. These teams are capable of working on several different aircraft and they can transform any aircraft into a mobile critical care unit (Fig. 6) [1].

CCAT team nurses can make a vital difference in the airborne environment, combining their critical care competence with knowledge of flight physiology to enhance patient outcomes [6]. Regarding flight physiology, one must keep in mind the nine stressors of flight: hypoxia, fatigue, changes in barometric pressure, effects of gravitational forces, noise, thermal stresses, vibration, fluid redistribution, and dehydration [8]. Deployed medical teams provide essential care in the field and depend on rapidly evacuating patients in stabilized rather than stable condition [9].

Preparing critically ill patients for movement to another medical facility takes a great deal of coordination. Just as the outgoing shift of hospital nurses reports on patients to nurses on the incoming shift, EMEDS nurses report on patients being transitioned to CCAT teams. Many patients are brought into the ER with their body armor and weapons. Nurses must ensure that patients are transported with their belongings. However, they must pay close attention to the transport of any weapons because weapons are not allowed in the open bay on the aircraft and must be secured in a locked container. In addition, nurses have to check that patients have an adequate supply of all medications and drips to cover possible rerouting of the aircraft and delayed arrival at the medical facility. Finally, all inpatient records and reports need to be sent to ensure a seamless transition of medical care and continuity of treatment.

**Trauma training**

To prepare for working in a war zone, military health care providers train in busy trauma centers all over the United States [3]. Not only do military providers benefit from caring for trauma patients in civilian settings but they also have the opportunity to train on high-tech simulated patients (eg, mannequins) in a controlled setting. This preparation enhances the capability of every medic who will encounter trauma in the combat zone [3].

*Clinical experiences*

At 0230 the call came in. A patient who had a severe gunshot wound was en route to the medical facility. The patient was hypotensive and tachycardic at the scene, where he had sustained an AK-47 gunshot wound to the lower leg. Blood loss was significant. When he arrived in the trauma room, he still had the intravenous (IV) fluid running that was started in the field, and his blood pressure had improved, although he was still tachycardic. During a primary medical survey, a blood-soaked field dressing on his lower

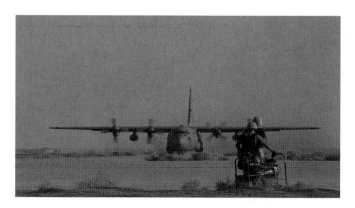

Fig. 6. C-130 takeoff from Tallil Air Base, Iraq.

calf was removed. Underneath the dressing, a large portion of calf muscle was blown out, leaving a gaping wound with small capillary bleeding.

A second urgent call came into the trauma room. Another gunshot injury was rolling through the ER doors. This patient was brought into the treatment facility by his buddies, who had witnessed the injury. The patient's left arm showed an obvious deformity with a small circular entry wound. Radiographs confirmed a shattered radius and ulnar, with displaced fractures and scattered bone fragments, and a 45-caliber bullet in the soft tissue.

### Center for Sustainment of Trauma and Readiness Skills

Were these casualties due to sniper fire in Baghdad? A firefight in Afghanistan? Guess again. These wounds were sustained by civilians in St. Louis, Missouri. These are just two real-life cases I experienced during a rotation at St. Louis University Hospital with the Center for Sustainment of Trauma and Readiness Skills (C-STARS) program. In the C-STARS program, military medics are seamlessly integrated into the trauma service of the medical center. Military physicians and midlevel providers serve as house staff on the trauma service, and nurses work in all critical care areas. Emergency medical technicians perform in the ER and on ambulances. Military medics at all levels have ample opportunities to participate in several procedures in the trauma room, ICUs, and the OR. (Incidentally, "medic" is a term of endearment and a label worn proudly by most military health care providers, including doctors, nurses, emergency medical technicians, and other allied health care members.) This program provides medics an authentic and meaningful exposure to significant trauma care, thus preparing them for trauma-related injuries that they are likely to see in the EMEDS.

C-STARS trainees at the St. Louis University School of Medicine also sharpened their skills in simulation laboratory exercises conducted in a state-of-the-art simulation laboratory. Mannequins representing patients were programmed to respond to medical treatment (real IVs, oxygen, and medications) by either improving or decompensating. This training laboratory mimics a trauma room in an EMEDS unit to give trainees the look and feel of how they might be working when deployed. An important aspect of the training was orientation to EMEDS equipment, some of which is unique to this military environment.

### Deployment setting in Iraq

The EMEDS plus 25 to which I was assigned was part of the 407th AEG in Tallil, about 200 miles southeast of Baghdad (Fig. 7). The USAF integrates all facets of its available forces, Active Duty, Guard, and Reserve, into its war fighting plan. As a traditional Air National Guardsman, I was stationed with active duty air force personnel in Iraq. Although I was the only member of

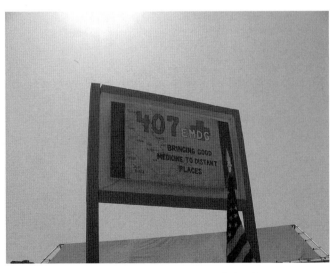

Fig. 7. 407th AEG EMEDS "motto" sign, Iraq.

the EMEDS direct patient care staff not to come from an active duty hospital, my integration into this active duty team was successful in every aspect.

While I was working in the EMEDS in Iraq, my clinical experiences varied day to day. Assigned as a nurse practitioner in the ER, I worked with my collaborating physician to provide sick call, which involved urgent and emergent care for all personnel assigned to the base or within our geographic treatment zone (Fig. 8). The clinical situations ranged from coughs and colds to mass casualties with critically injured patients. Our EMEDS had two ambulances that met the army dust-off choppers at their landing zone close to the EMEDS facility (Figs. 9 and 10). The ambulances were also used to transport critically injured patients to the flight line or tarmac, for transfer to and from awaiting aircraft. We were very lucky that our EMEDS module was connected to a trailer with bathrooms for staff and patients. My background in critical care and my experience as a clinical nurse specialist in dialysis and transplantation became valuable when a continuous veno-venous hemodialysis (CVVHD) program was being established in one of the regional theater hospitals in Baghdad. I worked with the nurses by e-mail and phone because this CVVHD machine happened to be one I had used to train ICU nurses in the past. I was able to provide them with some expertise by developing some training materials as they were getting started.

### Patient populations in the combat zone

Working in the ER of the EMEDS gave me the opportunity to care for people from all branches of the armed services, in addition to Department of Defense civilian personnel, local civilian workers, coalition forces, and locals with emergent medical situations. One example of the last was a local 8 year-old girl who had been bitten by a venomous snake [10]. When she arrived, her condition was critical and deteriorating quickly. With her mother and translator, who was an English teacher in the Iraqi school system, by her side around the clock, she received the best medical care that the USAF could offer and made a full recovery. This example underscores the importance of health care providers' cultural competence. The support from her family and community was tremendous. The staff at the EMEDS became local heroes, but the real hero was the little girl who braved more than 2 weeks of aggressive medical treatment without any complaints. This clinical situation provided some firsthand experience with the surrounding community, whose acceptance of our work was gratifying.

### Clinical situations in the combat zone

*Situation #1*

Within the first few days of arriving in Iraq and before I had adjusted to the hot temperatures of the desert, I experienced my first mass casualty

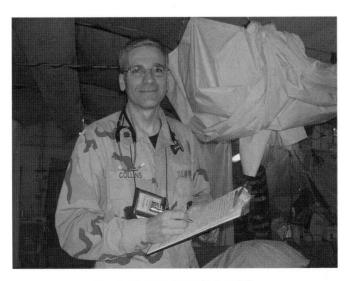

Fig. 8. Working in ER in EMEDS.

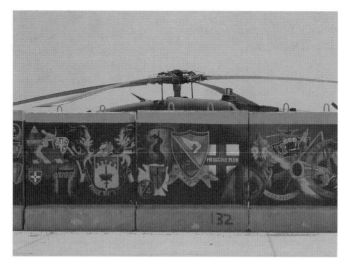

Fig. 9. Awaiting army dust-off chopper.

alert. Two hours earlier, I had left work to go to the air base library to write a paper for a course I was taking at University of Massachusetts, when I heard the commotion of trucks and choppers overhead. Whether from gut feeling or just curiosity, I was drawn to return to the EMEDS unit to see what was happening. Indeed, preparations were underway to prepare for mass casualties. The ER was being transformed before my eyes from a four-bed evaluation station into an open bay trauma room. The teamwork and precision of these preparations were only outdone by the care delivered when the patients arrived.

Because most of the trauma included shattered bones requiring a high level of expertise, the orthopedic surgeon was always in high demand.

Our trauma training was now fully activated to perform primary and secondary surveys rapidly. Although the environment was new for all members of the health care team, we performed our tasks like a well-practiced sports team. Blood was drawn, spun, and analyzed. Radiographs from stretchers were taken, one after another. Multiple patients were simultaneously and rapidly intubated and stabilized. Burn dressings were applied and vasoactive medications infused. Several

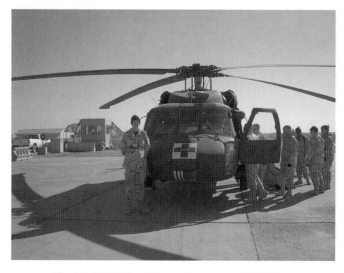

Fig. 10. Supporting army medic chopper, Tallil, Iraq.

patients were admitted to the ICU. Almost immediately, the flight surgeons began coordinating the intricate aeromedical evacuation system. This system ensured that critical care staff was available to provide complex medical care en route to seriously injured troops as they were being transported to more definitive care at a regional medical facility, usually in Germany.

One memory that will never leave me is carrying the stretcher of a critically injured soldier into the open bay of a C-17 cargo plane, because just the night before he and other critically injured troops had first rolled through the ER doors and had been resuscitated. These troops were departing while on ventilators and vasoactive medications. A detailed report was given to the CCAT team that took over the care of these patients. Two critical nurses helped to ensure that all equipment was working properly and secured. I waited in the ambulance on the flight line until the plane became airborne. If the plane had to abort its mission, we had to be prepared to transport patients back to the EMEDS ICU quickly.

*Situation #2*

The door of the ER was flung open, and a fellow airman uttered a dramatic cry for help. Several medics working in the ER ran out to assist him. Moments later they rushed through the door carrying a litter (stretcher) with a critically injured airman. The ER was instantly set into motion for transformation. The patient was conscious but had significant upper body burns with possible upper airway damage. The ER team rapidly sedated and intubated the patient and began fluid resuscitation before he was transferred to the ICU (Fig. 11). This airman urgently needed to be transferred to more definitive care for upper body and inhalation burns, so the flight surgeon initiated coordination of the CCAT team transfer.

*Situation #3*

Another mass casualty alert and we prepared for the arrival of patients. Some medics at the scene relayed that a critically injured airman was pinned in wreckage and was being resuscitated in the field. He arrived in dire condition with shattered legs, and the extent of his orthopedic injuries was visually devastating. Another two patients were brought in with multiple injuries, but our first patient was in the most critical condition. The physical layout of the EMEDS was solidified as this patient was intubated and

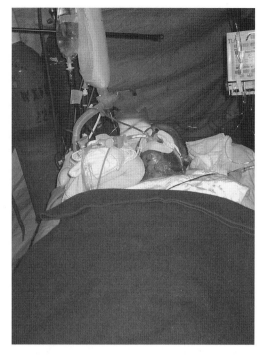

Fig. 11. Burn patient in 407th EMEDS ICU.

resuscitated in the ER and then wheeled on his stretcher 30 feet back into the OR. The OR team worked with great urgency to prepare all the equipment and supplies necessary to save this man's life. The orthopedic surgeon spent several hours attempting to salvage the patient's badly damaged legs. The OR nurse and nurse anesthetist worked feverishly, providing blood transfusions and fluid resuscitation and maintaining a sense of order in a chaotic situation. After extensive surgery to stabilize and reduce his multiple fractures, the patient was transferred to the ICU.

In the ICU, he continued to receive outstanding care. Although his multiple fractures and internal injuries had been addressed in the OR, the struggle for his recovery continued. The flight surgeons coordinated his CCAT team flight to Landstuhl Regional Medical Center in Germany for continuation of his care and recovery. During his recovery, this patient was followed closely by a group of nurses and providers who had been "adopted" by the patient's friends and fellow service members for their work in saving his life. His progress was sporadically reported to us throughout our deployment. Hearing from a wounded patient for whom a medic has cared is a humbling and rewarding experience. It is immensely satisfying to see a patient make progress from an initially dire situation. With great pride and hope, we later read a Christmas greeting card from this patient, with a photo of him standing on both legs at Walter Reed Hospital. In the tumult of the ER, a medic has only one focus: to save a life. Knowing that one's efforts have paid off is professionally and personally rewarding.

*Situation #4*

One challenge of working in a deployed military situation is that one never knows who or what clinical situation will come through the door. A case in point was a critically ill child brought to the front gate of the base. She had a high fever and respiratory distress that called for immediate medical intervention. A child in an EMEDS unit can pose a problem on the best of days. Military medics are accustomed to working on adults, but caring for children requires a different mind-set and specific pediatric equipment. However, this life-and-death situation spurred us on to improvise and create supplies to work on such a small patient. With some ingenuity and teamwork, the improvised supplies allowed us to deliver outstanding care that resulted in the successful management of the clinical situation. This 1-year-old infant had clearly been septic, with an extremely high fever and respiratory distress. Her clinical situation improved with antibiotics and antipyretics. The source that contributed to her infection was identified by telemedicine, whereby a radiologist stationed at another base identified an abdominal tumor.

**Summary**

Military members who carry a stethoscope are proud to be called "medic." They all accept their role as bringing good medicine to a difficult place for well-deserving warriors. EMEDS doctors and nurses must always be prepared for the worst-case scenario, with no notice, and multiple casualties [11]. During my career, I have forged many strong relationships while caring for patients in the most difficult of circumstances, and have grown to appreciate the contributions of a well-organized and dedicated group of individuals. No matter how difficult the environment and circumstances, this EMEDS team provided the best possible medical care to all who passed through its door (Fig. 12).

The distinct thumping of the rotary blades of a military helicopter is recognizable from a distance, and as it approaches, the cadence of those blades conjures up memories of the mission and the purpose of our work as deployed medics. In the M*A*S*H series, just the word "choppers" over the loudspeaker set medics into motion to care for the military's most valuable assets. The sound of choppers today still provokes this feeling in all medics who have served in a combat zone. The rewards for medics are deep and rich: knowing firsthand that the care provided in the most critical of situations can translate into the

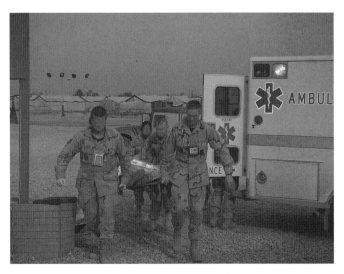

Fig. 12. Bringing the wounded into the ER of EMEDS.

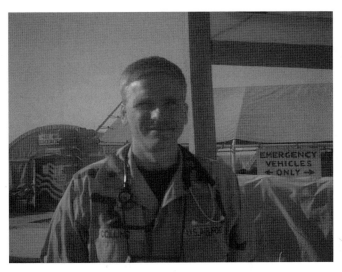

Fig. 13. Outside 407th AEG EMEDS.

successful recovery of a fellow warrior. Nurses in deployed settings bring a great deal of knowledge and clinical competence to their work, whether in an EMEDS unit or as part of a CCAT team. Capturing the rich experience and lessons learned is of great importance as nurses continue to provide patient care on the front lines. Success means being prepared to do one's job in the most austere environment and against incredible obstacles, while always remaining flexible (Fig. 13).

## References

[1] Callander BD. After M*A*S*H. Air Force Magazine 2004;87(12):66–70.

[2] Skelton PA, Droege L, Carlisle MT. EMEDS and SPEARR teams: United States Air Force ready responders. Crit Care Nurs Clin North Am 2003;15: 201–12.

[3] Taylor GP. Statement of Lieutenant General George Taylor Jr., Air Force Surgeon General before the House Armed Services Committee, Personnel Subcommittee on the Fiscal Year 2006 Medical Program. 19 October 2005. Available at: http://armedservices.house.gov/comdocs/schedules/2005.htm.

[4] Darr L, Binder J, Vivian TN, et al. Air Force Medical Services concept of operations for Expeditionary Medical Support (EMEDS)/Air Force Theater Hospital (AFTH) system. Available at: www.brooksidepress.org.

[5] Dunn WJ. Dental emergency rates at an Expeditionary Medical Support facility supporting Operation Enduring Freedom. Mil Med 2004;169(5):349–53.

[6] Pierce PF, Evers KG. Global presence: USAF aeromedical evacuation and critical care transport. Crit Care Nurs Clin North Am 2003;15:221–31.

[7] Air Force Medical Services concept of operations for aeromedical evacuation. 14 July 2000. Available at: http://www.brooksidepress.org/ Products/OperationalMedicine/DATA/operationalmed/ OperationalSettings/Air%20Force/AFMSCONOPs.htm.

[8] Schmelz JO, Bridges EJ, Duong DN, et al. Care of the critically ill patient in a military unique environment: a program of research. Crit Care Nurs Clin North Am 2003;15:171–81.

[9] Carlton PK. New millennium, new mind-set, the Air Force Medical Service in the air expeditionary era. Aerospace Power Journal 2000;15(4):8–13. Available at: http://www.airpower.maxwell.af.mil/ airchronicles/apjc.html.

[10] Svan JH. Iraq puts a medic's training to test. Stars and Stripes, Pacific edition 2004. August 1, 2004. Available at: http://www.stripesonline.com/article. asp?section=104&article=22629&archive=true.

[11] Chrenkoff A. Two nations in one: a roundup of the past two weeks' good news from Iraq. Editorial from The Wall Street Journal. Available at: http://www. opinionjournal.com/extra/?id=110005801.

**ELSEVIER
SAUNDERS**

Crit Care Nurs Clin N Am 20 (2008) 13–22

**CRITICAL CARE
NURSING CLINICS
OF NORTH AMERICA**

# Skill Set Requirements for Nurses Deployed with an Expeditionary Medical Unit Based on Lessons Learned

John J. Whitcomb, PhD, RN, CCRN, CDR, NC, USN[a],*,
Kimberly J. Newell, RN, MSN, CCRN, CNS, CDR, NC, USN[b]

[a]*Naval Medical Center Portsmouth, 620 John Paul Jones Circle,
Portsmouth, VA 23708, USA*
[b]*Naval Hospital Camp Pendleton, Box 555191, Camp Pendleton, CA 92055, USA*

Based in Kuwait 3 years apart, the authors recount how nurses and corps staff, along with their physician counterparts, came together to form well-run medical facilities under adverse circumstances. Their respective hospitals became competent organizations because of specific formulas for success, along with preparation, identification of required skill sets, and making improvements based on experience. This article describes the training of medical, nursing, and corps staff, the facilities and resources required for managing casualties, and some of the more commonly encountered combat injuries and conditions.

* Corresponding author.
*E-mail address:* john.whitcomb@med.navy.mil
(J.J. Whitcomb).

## Camp Coyote, Kuwait, 2003

In February 2003, the 1st Force Service Support Group (FSSG), 4th Health Services Battalion (HSB) was activated in support of Operation Iraqi Freedom. Active-duty health care professionals and mobilized reservists with various health care backgrounds combined forces to form a cohesive combat-support hospital located approximately 30 miles from the Iraq border, at Camp Coyote in Kuwait. This unit, the 4th HSB, was designed to deploy to an area of conflict where it would receive and treat war causalities. Regardless of the mission, and although segments of the support group had yet to arrive, this advanced-party team had the means and "can-do spirit" that allowed them to be ready to receive casualties within days of its arrival in Kuwait.

## Brief historical review

On the same ground where Desert Storm occurred, the 4th HSB was set up to provide emergency resuscitation and definitive surgery, saving life and limb, and to offer general medical care under field and combat conditions. Medical specialties that deployed with the 4th HSB included trauma, thoracic surgery, orthopedic surgery, psychiatry, ophthalmology, general surgery, internal medicine, and family practice. The nursing staff specialties included critical care, obstetric/gynecologic, pediatric, and medical-surgical nurses, family nurse practitioners, and nurse administrators

0899-5885/08/$ - see front matter. Published by Elsevier Inc.
doi:10.1016/j.ccell.2007.10.009

*ccnursing.theclinics.com*

with varying degrees of clinical experience. The Hospital Corps staff (composed of enlisted personnel who perform patient care activities under the direction of licensed providers) consisted of individuals trained as paramedics, general duty corps staff, psychiatric technicians, pharmacy technicians, x-ray technicians, and independent duty corpsmen. Independent duty corpsmen function similarly to physician assistants. Support services included laboratory, x-ray, pharmacy, administration, and chaplaincy. Security for the entire camp was provided by the Marine Corps.

The 4th HSB was tasked to provide the services of a surgical hospital (echelon II), receiving casualties from forward deployed units. Echelons start with the simplest care closest to the battle zone (level I), where someone may put on his or her own dressing or have a comrade do so (a procedure known as "buddy aid"). If possible, this event is followed by a trip to the Battalion Aid Station, Forward Resuscitation Surgical Support unit, or Shock Trauma Platoon. At these stations, a physician, independent duty corpsman, or nurse provides first aid or advanced trauma life support, preserving life or limb. Given available transportation and a favorable battlefield scenario, ground transport or Blackhawk helicopter transport transfers the casualty to a level II facility, such as the 4th HSB, for stabilization. The casualty may move on

in a matter of hours or, if conditions dictate, may be retained for 24 to 48 hours. The next echelon (level III) is the combat zone fleet hospital or the hospital ship. Both air and ground transportation are used to move a patient to this echelon of care, as dictated by the tactical situation, the presence or absence of enemy air threats, and/or overwhelming troop movements. The final destination for definitive care is a facility outside the combat area, such as a medical treatment facility (MTF) in the continental United States [1]. "MTF" is the military term designating clinics, hospitals, and other health care facilities found in the civilian world.

The 4th HSB consisted of a receiving area (triage) that led to two operating rooms that adjoined two ICUs, each with a capacity for 12 patients. There were three wards, each with the ability to hold 30 patients. An outpatient area treated injuries that did not need inpatient care. The facility offered services including radiology, a blood bank, a small laboratory, and a pharmacy. Its purpose was to stabilize patients and transport them within 24 hours to a higher echelon level of care in Kuwait (Figs. 1–3).

### Staff assignment, education, and training

The Bureau of Naval Personnel assigns military members to specific operational platforms

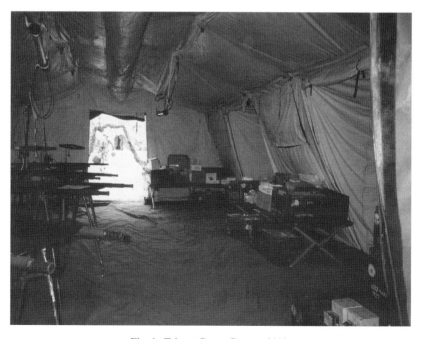

Fig. 1. Triage, Camp Coyote, 2003.

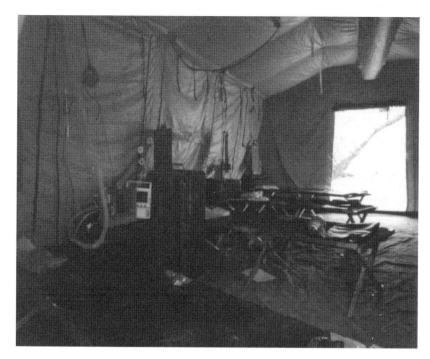

Fig. 2. ICU set-up, Camp Coyote, 2003.

(ie, hospital ships, fleet hospitals and FSSG units), with their primary duty station being an MTF [2]. For the 1st FSSG, Navy military personnel are mobilized from the Naval Medical Center San Diego, California and Naval Reserve Unit, 4th HSB. The 4th HSB also was supported by individual augmentees, military members assigned according to their clinical specialties and the unit's

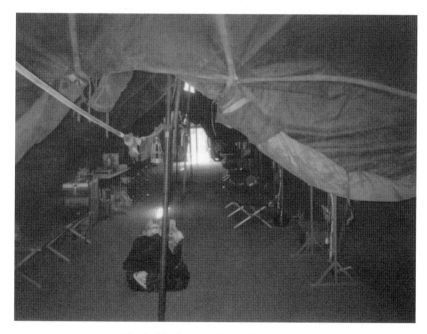

Fig. 3. Ward set-up, Camp Coyote, 2003.

needs. Total personnel for this unit consisted of 30 nurses, 66 corps staff, and 20 physicians. These numbers increased or decreased based on mission requirements (Fig. 4).

The Bureau of Navy Medicine and the commanding officers of the local supporting MTFs continually assess readiness needs and train medical personnel for their assignments accordingly. Typically, preparation for serving with fleet hospitals, FSSGs, and other ground units consists of field training with the Marines in a setting similar to the actual austere environments to which trainees will or may deploy. While serving with the Fleet Marine Force, hospital corps staff train to care for the warfighter on the battlefield. Physicians and nurses attend courses that prepare them to care for trauma patients. The Trauma Nursing Core Course (TNCC) is offered at the three main Navy MTFs and is required for all Navy nurses.

The TNCC is a fundamental course that enhances cognitive skills, sharpens technical skills, and provides a foundation for future learning to nurses actively involved in caring for injured patients. The TNCC is presented in lectures and in six psychomotor-skill stations. The focus is on airway management, spinal immobilization, initial assessment, multiple trauma intervention, and splinting. These foundational sessions allow participants to develop and enhance their practical skills using mannequins and live models. The sessions enable nurses to become well acquainted with emergency situations and expose them to the use of the appropriate equipment. Participants learn to assess the patient, identify life-threatening emergencies, and identify and prioritize other injuries. A provider manual reinforces and supplements lectures and lessons in psychomotor skills. Each aspect of trauma is discussed using common basic themes: etiology, mechanism of injury and concurrent injuries, anatomy and physiology, pathophysiology (as a basis for key signs and symptoms), nursing care, patient education, and triage. Following completion of the course, both theoretical and practical knowledge are assessed formally by written and practical examination.

Physicians attend the Advanced Trauma Life Support Course, which teaches them to assess the patient's condition rapidly and accurately, to resuscitate and stabilize the patient according to priority, to determine if the patient's needs exceed a facility's capabilities, to arrange appropriately for the patient's definitive care, and to ensure that optimal care is provided. Another course that is available, developed by the Society of Critical Care Medicine, is the Fundamentals of Critical Care Course. This 2-day course is designed for

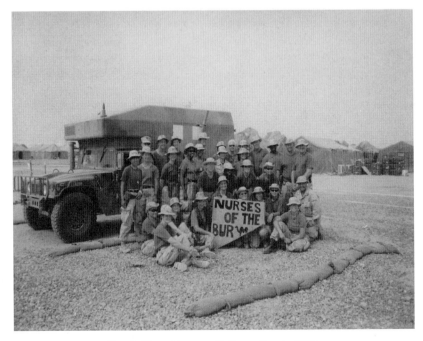

Fig. 4. Nurse Corps staff, Camp Coyote, 2003.

nurses and physicians who are not intensivists in critical care. It offers skills stations, lectures, and guidance for decision making during the initial hours of management of critically ill patients.

## Assessment of personnel

Because providers have different backgrounds and experience, they are assessed by the 4th HSB leadership team to determine how best to use their skills and to determine who needs training in specific assessment and skill sets. The first author was named the unit's Director for Nursing Care. He managed the clinical aspects of nursing care. Another senior nurse managed the administrative nursing functions. The Director for Nursing Care divided the nursing personnel into four groups, each containing at least two critical care nurses and corps staff trained in the Fleet Marine Force or as paramedics. Personnel then were placed in groups based on level of expertise to ensure that no one team had all the expertise. A team leader was identified to orient, train, and manage personnel in patient care. This training had to occur within a few days of arrival because of the imminent influx of causalities. This team approach proved highly successful, because those who had no trauma or critical care experience felt supported by being grouped with those who had experience (Fig. 5).

In preparation for the receipt of patients, the Director for Nursing Care and his team leaders provided personnel with refresher training, using the TNCC curriculum coupled with the team leaders' past experiences. They "got back to the basics" of nursing care. They assembled and tested medical equipment and held classes to discuss the plan of action with the threat of air or ground attack and the possible use of chemical or biologic agents. Most personnel had been trained previously, to some extent, to respond to these threats; in the field, however, such threats were compounded by the intense heat and never-ending sand storms, which created a heightened sense of anxiety. A matter of great concern was that many of these individuals had never witnessed trauma or been in a real-time combat zone. Therefore, discussing possible scenarios was extremely valuable in providing anticipatory guidance. Encouraging the staff to talk to and support each other also was extremely helpful to them. Such discussions were key to the prevention of posttraumatic stress disorder (PTSD) among

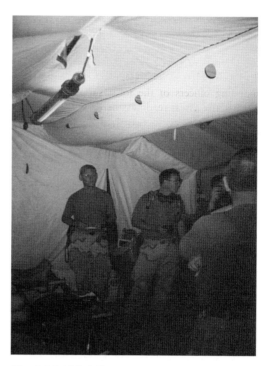

Fig. 5. Multidisciplinary rounds, Camp Coyote, 2003.

health care professionals who treat patients with combat trauma.

## Posttraumatic stress disorder

PTSD is commonly associated with soldiers plagued by horrific memories of battle. It can also be found among those who treat injured soldiers. Experiencing or witnessing a frightening event that arouses intense feelings of fear, helplessness, or horror sets the stage for PTSD. The trauma has such a strong impact that the victim cannot shake the experience and relives the painful emotions associated with it. Sudden flashbacks may occur. Other symptoms include an exaggerated startle reflex, sleep disturbances and nightmares, irritability, angry outbursts, difficulty concentrating, hallucinations, sexual dysfunction, and an inability to speak about the tragedy [3]. The austere environment and extreme weather conditions in Kuwait contributed to provider stress and anxiety, as did the use of equipment that was not as sophisticated as that to which staff were accustomed. Temperatures reached well into the 110°F range, creating concern for personnel safety. Extreme temperatures also made running simple laboratory tests difficult. Sand storms raged without warning. Discussing threats and listening to staff concerns about the capabilities of the equipment, the working environment, and the weather prepared them for many eventualities and helped them cope with anxiety. Staff were encouraged to have open discussions among themselves and to support one another, an effective strategy that was used many times during this deployment.

### Patient care and lessons learned

On April 15, 2003, the 4th HSB began receiving casualties caused by heat exposure, explosive devices, gunshots, and motor vehicle accidents. The providers at Camp Coyote also were responsible for treating illnesses unique to the country and for attending to the day-to-day medical needs of the troops. In all, from April 15 until June 25, the staff treated more than 200 casualties. It was amazing to see the staff in action, working as a team, mentoring and supporting one another day and night. Each individual knew that he or she could call on a fellow shipmate in time of need. The formula for success included the staff's positive, "can-do" attitude and their strong nursing education in the areas of trauma management and critical thinking. Past experience and key concepts from the TNCC and advanced cardiac life support courses also prepared the nurses for their wartime experience.

Navy Nurse Corps officers led by example. They never asked a lower-ranking officer or enlisted person to do anything they would not do themselves. Selecting the right people for the right job was highly effective, because those with more experience provided education and leadership and knew when it was appropriate to intervene or support other team members. Finally, the nursing leadership of the 4th HSB planned for the worst-case scenarios, and this planning prepared them to be resilient and flexible throughout the deployment. Personnel understood that plans could change at a moment's notice. The term "day off" did not apply. When casualties arrived, everyone joined in to support those on duty.

Lessons learned were that more real-time hands-on training would be desirable in future deployments. Also prior training on the equipment to be used in the field, along with gaining experience at civilian trauma centers, would greatly benefit those who had never treated a trauma patient.

### Expeditionary Medical Facility Kuwait, 2006

In the 3 years between the first and second author's deployments, the Navy's medical support in the Kuwaiti theater of operations transitioned from an echelon II to an echelon III facility and was relocated from the northern part of the country to the southern part. Like the Camp Coyote facility in 2003, Detachment B of Expeditionary Medical Facility (EMF) Kuwait in Camp Arifjan in 2006 was a melting pot for both Nurse Corps officers and Hospital Corps staff. The 40 nursing staff members assigned to the Inpatient Nursing Department deployed from 12 MTFs, including ambulatory clinics, small and medium-sized community hospitals, and large tertiary-care teaching facilities. Within these facilities, staff had performed various functions and represented assorted clinical services: administrative, bedside clinician, clinical nurse specialist, and division officer (unit manager). These individuals came from dental, medical/surgical, maternal/child, pediatric, emergency room, intensive care, and post-anesthesia care environments. Although few knew each other before coming together as a full EMF detachment in March 2006, the diverse group, like the 4th HSB, quickly became a cohesive unit that learned to capitalize on one another's strengths (Fig. 6).

The first of two waves of medical personnel arrived in late February 2006 and received turnover information from the outgoing detachment. Three weeks later, the second wave arrived and turned over with the remainder of the outgoing detachment along with the first wave in the EMF's detachment—their new "shipmates." With less than 2 weeks of orientation and turnover, the group assumed the reins of a four-bed casualty-receiving (CASREC) unit, a four-bed ICU, and 24 medical/surgical beds that could be expanded to a total of 44 beds for a mass-casualty situation. The second author was assigned as head of the 40 staff members and 44 beds of the Inpatient Nursing Department. Staff were divided into four teams, each consisting of four nurses and five corps staff. To capitalize on nurses' advanced knowledge and skills, one nurse who had emergency experience and one nurse who had intensive care experience were assigned to each team. Low numbers of ICU patients at the time provided an opportunity for the staff to expand their knowledge and skills by rotating between the three clinical areas. Teams spent 2 weeks on the ward and 2 weeks in CASREC. They then returned to the ward for 2 weeks, after which they worked in

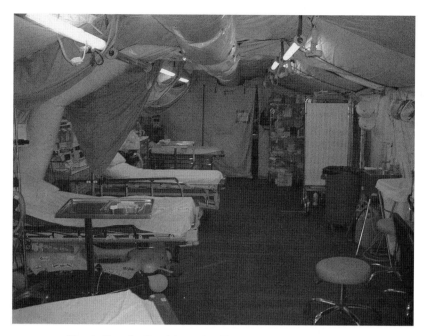

Fig. 6. Casualty Receiving, US Military Hospital, Kuwait, 2006.

the ICU for 2 weeks. If there were no patients in the ICU, the nurse would cross-train in the post-anesthesia care unit or the operating room or would serve as an additional nurse in CASREC or on the ward, as needed. Ancillary services included laboratory, pharmacy, and radiology. Medical and dental specialties available during the 6-month rotation included anesthesia, general surgery, gynecology, orthopedics, internal medicine, cardiology, gastroenterology, infectious disease, pulmonology, pediatrics, psychiatry, dentistry, and oral surgery. Gastroenterologists, infectious disease specialists, and pediatricians were deployed as general internists, but their respective specialty skills proved to be quite useful.

As noted in Fig. 7, the main hospital building consisted of five interconnecting sets of modular tents placed parallel to one another. One main perpendicular passageway through the center of each tent connected neighboring tents with one another. Additional tents housed administration, communications, supplies, the armory, and operations.

### Assessment of personnel

The second author rapidly realized that an assessment of the knowledge and skill of the recently arrived new personnel was required. This assessment was accomplished in three ways.

Initially, to provide an opportunity for all staff to learn a little bit about each other, brief self-introductions were made at a staff meeting. This author and her senior enlisted leader then met individually with each of the staff members to learn more about their personal and clinical backgrounds, strengths, and goals for the 6-month deployment. She then developed and conducted an educational needs assessment based on the current and future conditions for the expected patient population.

To assess the educational needs of the staff properly, it was important to determine the expected patient population for the next 6 months. A review of the admission International Classification of Diseases (edition 9) codes for the prior months of February and March revealed that chest pain, appendicitis/status-post appendectomy, hernia/status-post hernia repair, and cellulitis were the top four admission diagnoses. Realizing that the knowledge and skill levels of the staff were varied and that there was a potential for receiving high-acuity patients, she assessed the need for staff training to care for these possible high-volume or high-risk diagnoses. She also assessed equipment-training needs for these higher-acuity conditions.

A review of the results from a staff educational needs survey revealed that they had little to no knowledge or experience caring for critically ill or

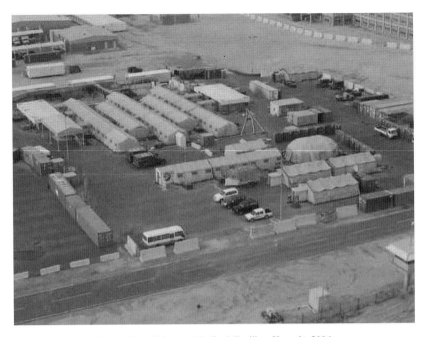

Fig. 7. Expeditionary Medical Facility, Kuwait, 2006.

critically injured patients or in using the equipment seen in a fleet hospital ICU. Working with a fellow clinical nurse specialist, a training plan was developed that included a combination of hour-long continuing education lectures, 10- to 15-minute in-services, skills laboratories, and a plan to perform an educational needs postassessment toward the end of the 6-month deployment. On average, one nursing continuing education lecture and one or two in-services were scheduled each week, in addition to a total of six skills laboratories specifically targeting the topics with the lowest mean knowledge and/or experience scores.

Several months later, the same educational needs survey was redistributed for postassessment purposes. A review of the results revealed the items with the lowest increase in knowledge from the pre- to the postassessment were care of the patient in cardiorespiratory arrest and care of the pulmonary/respiratory patient, probably because, throughout the 6-month deployment, only one patient required cardiopulmonary resuscitation, and only a few had reactive airway disease or pneumonia. Items with the highest increase in knowledge from the pre- to the post-assessment were use of the Alaris MedSystem III infusion pump (Cardinal Health, Dublin, Ohio), cellulitis, care of the patient with wounds, hernias/status-post

hernia repair, and ventilator concepts (eg, modes, settings, weaning). Incidentally, the Alaris MedSystem III infusion pump is the only intravenous infusion pump authorized for use in the military aeromedical evacuation system, but few Navy MTFs use this particular model as the primary pump for intravenous fluid infusion; therefore, in-services on this piece of equipment were needed. As stated previously, cellulitis and hernia/status-post hernia repair were two of the top three admission diagnoses during February and March, and this trend continued through September. Therefore, the increase in knowledge directly reflects the experience acquired with this patient population during this deployment. Although the EMF only had one patient who required mechanical ventilation, this was the topic of one of the continuing education lectures provided by the pulmonologist, who also was certified as an intensivist.

Items with the lowest increase in experience from the pre- to the postassessment were intubation/extubation assistance and cardioversion. Throughout the deployment, only one patient required intubation. Because it was expected that the staff would care for patients requiring intubation, extubation, however, trauma airway management was one of the continuing education lectures provided by one of the EMF's nurse anesthetists.

Items with the highest increase in experience from the pre- to the postassessment were hernia/status-post hernia repair, use of the Welch Allyn Propaq Monitor (Welch Allyn, Beaverton, Oregon), nephrolithiasis, and care of the postoperative patient. Because of its portability and air-worthiness (ie, its capability to function during air transport), the Welch Allyn Propaq Monitor is the cardiac monitoring system found in the fleet hospital system. The EMF used it in the ICU and during ground and aeromedical evacuation. Because of the absence of a central monitoring system, and in lieu of telemetry monitoring, it also was used on the ward for patients requiring cardiac monitoring. Like the Alaris MedSystem III, few Navy MTFs use this equipment as the primary mode of cardiac monitoring. Although data are unavailable at this time regarding the number of patients admitted with nephrolithiasis, it is estimated that two to four patients per month were admitted with this diagnosis. As with changes in knowledge, changes in experience directly reflected the patient population served during the deployment.

Some would view this 6-month experience as a group of individuals in the right place at the right time; others would view this same group as being in the wrong place at the wrong time. As it turns out, the average patient cared for by Detachment B of EMF Kuwait was low acuity, primarily because the location was too far away from the "front-line" to receive combat casualties. This level III facility in southern Kuwait provided garrison-level care but also was a receiving facility for patients requiring specialty services from throughout the Persian Gulf region. This low-acuity population was not the case for Detachment B's predecessors—Detachment A—or successors—Detachment C—who experienced at least one mass-casualty event of higher-acuity patients during each deployment. A forward-deployed level III facility, such as this EMF, would expect to care for more and higher-acuity patients than the second author's detachment did during this particular 6-month deployment.

Ideally, in planning for the staffing of these facilities, 25% of the inpatient nursing department staff should have at least 1 year of emergency nursing experience, 25% should have at least 1 year of ICU experience, and the remaining 50% should have a combination of medical, surgical, and/or psychiatric experience. Because staff are rotated through all clinical areas, and because a primary responsibility of Navy Nurse Corps officers is to train corps staff, at least 75% of the nurses should be certified in both advanced cardiac life support and TNCC. Because of the operational tempo and the determination to deploy everyone once before any one person was required to return for a second deployment, recommendations regarding clinical experience could not always be met. In this case, any exposure to medical, surgical, mental health, intensive care, or emergency nursing that can be obtained before deployment is beneficial.

## Summary

The authors, in describing their respective experiences in Kuwait, have shown that recognition of required skills and appropriate education provided before deployment is vital to the successful operation of echelon II and III medical facilities. In addition, they demonstrate that the experience gained and the training provided during deployment are essential for optimal outcomes in current and future missions. Because of changes in stability of the area, a better geographic location within Kuwait, a less-acute patient load in general, and improved medical equipment in the Kuwaiti theater of operations, the 2006 mission was able to assess needs systematically, provide formal training, and evaluate the success or failure of that training more easily than could their colleagues from earlier deployments.

Despite their different circumstances, the authors took advantage of every possible opportunity to prepare, train, and support their staff members by expanding their knowledge and skills to provide the best possible care to those warriors entrusted to their care while still in theater.

## Acknowledgments

The authors wish to acknowledge June Brockman, Medical Editor, Naval Medical Center, Portsmouth, Virginia, for her contributions in the preparation of this article. CDR Newell would like to acknowledge and thank CAPT Kriste Grau, NC, USN and all the nurses and corpsmen of the Inpatient Nursing Department who embraced coming together in an austere environment, who never backed down from a challenge, and who made the deployment as enjoyable as it was. Finally, they both thank their spouses and families for their unwavering support during the deployments.

## References

[1] Hrezo R. Navy nurse anesthetists at Fleet Hospital Five. The Desert Shield/Storm experience. Crit Care Nurs Clin North Am 2003;15(2):213–20.

[2] Boren D, Forbus R, Bibeau P, et al. Managing critical care casualties on the Navy's hospital ships. Crit Care Nurs Clin North Am 2003;15(2):184–91.

[3] Fagan N, Freme K. Confronting posttraumatic stress disorder. Nursing 2004;34(2):52–3.

ELSEVIER
SAUNDERS

Crit Care Nurs Clin N Am 20 (2008) 23–29

CRITICAL CARE
NURSING CLINICS
OF NORTH AMERICA

# The Synergy Model at Work in a Military ICU in Iraq

Mary E. Freyling, RN, MS, CCRN, CCNS, LTC, AN, USA[a,*],
Karen S. Kesten, RN, MSN, CCRN, PCCN, CCNS[b],
Janie Heath, PhD, APRN-BC, ANP, ACNP[c]

[a]Tripler Army Medical Center, Surgical Product Line, 1 Jarrett White Road, Honolulu, HI 96859, USA
[b]Georgetown University School of Nursing & Health Studies, 3700 Reservoir Road, Washington, DC 20057, USA
[c]Medical College of Georgia School of Nursing, 997 Saint Sebastian Way, Augusta, GA 30912, USA

While starting the American Association of Critical-Care Nurses (AACN) application process for the Acute and Critical Care Clinical Nurse Specialist (CCNS) examination, two unexpected hurdles occurred. First, the primary author (Lieutenant Colonel Freyling, who held the Army rank of Major (MAJ) during the occasion of this article) did not have all of the required 500 clinical hours in her master of science in nursing program and second, military orders arrived for her to deploy to Iraq. As an Army nurse who had a critical care background, she knew all things were possible even in the face of significant challenges. After a few phone calls, precepted clinical hours were arranged with an academic institution, and she was back on track to achieving her goal to become CCNS-certified, even if she was heading to Iraq.

## Overview of the American Association of Critical Care Nurses synergy model

Along with the surprise of life in the desert, MAJ Freyling found that AACN's synergy model served her well as she started to work in a military ICU in Iraq (Fig. 1). It was clear to her that effective nursing practice, whether providing direct patient care in the United States or in an ICU in Iraq, is demonstrated when care is centered around the needs and characteristics of patients. AACN's Synergy Model for Patient Care values patient-centered care and demonstrates that positive patient outcomes are achieved when the competencies of the nurse and the characteristics of the patient are matched to meet the needs of the patient [1]. There are eight characteristics in the synergy model that are unique for patients who experience critical events (Table 1). There are also eight competencies in the synergy model that are essential for nurses to have when providing patient care (Table 2). Increasingly, the literature supports that when patient characteristics and nurse competencies are matched, opportunities for optimal patient outcomes are enhanced [2]. The synergy model also includes different levels of care required to meet the needs of the patients ranging from high (level 1) to minimal (level 5) and levels of competency ranging from competent (level 1) to expert (level 5). In addition, the model includes three spheres of influence: those derived through the nurse's influence with patients and families, nurses, and health care systems [3].

The synergy model may provide a helpful framework for the multifaceted role of the nurse taking care of acutely and critically ill patients in a military field hospital. MAJ Freyling found daily encounters of presenting patient characteristics and nurse competencies demonstrated throughout her military assignment working in the field ICU and transporting patients to a larger military facility. Although many components of the synergy model occur simultaneously, four are highlighted. First, advocacy and moral agency

The views expressed in this manuscript are those of the authors and do not reflect the official policy or position of the Department of the Army, Department of Defense, or the United States Government.

* Corresponding author.
 *E-mail address:* beth.freyling@us.army.mil
(M.E. Freyling).

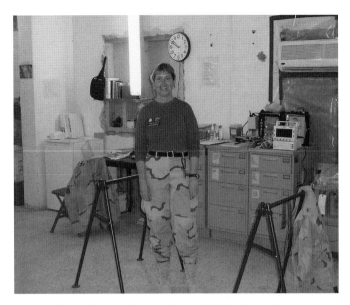

Fig. 1. Forward Surgical Team, ICU Section, in Iraq.

(a nurse competency) and vulnerability (a patient characteristic) are described for the care of an Arab female child with 45% burns from an improvised explosive device (IED) thrown into her front door. Then, diversity (a nurse competency denoting the ability to recognize the individuality of patients) [1], participation in care (a patient characteristic denoting engagement in aspects of care) [1], and resiliency (a patient characteristic denoting the ability to return to a prior level of functioning) [1] are described for the care of an Arab female who had traumatic brain injury from a vehicle-borne IED. These two cases demonstrate how characteristics fluctuate with a patient's condition and how nurse competencies, when linked synergistically, can improve the outcomes for patients requiring critical care in a military ICU in Iraq.

### Advocacy and moral agency: snapshot of competency in a military ICU in Iraq

Advocacy and moral agency is a nurse competency that can be defined as acting on the behalf of another to ensure that person's best interests are considered [1,4]. Several patient characteristics profit from the application of this competency. One that consistently manifested during MAJ Freyling's assignment was the patient characteristic of vulnerability, or the susceptibility to stressors that may affect outcomes adversely

[1,3]. Most trauma patients are vulnerable, as trauma is a stressor known to adversely affect outcomes. Complicate the stress of trauma with patients who are chemically paralyzed, sedated, in severe pain, or even comatose, and this alters their ability to participate in care and decision making [5]; thus there is a requirement of a higher level of competency for advocacy and moral agency by the nurse.

Vulnerability of Iraqi patients, in particular, also includes a language barrier. The inability to participate in care and decision making in the case of Iraqi patients is compounded by this communication deficit, and this can result in disjointed care [5]. An important role of the CCNS is to establish an environment that promotes ethical decision making and patient advocacy. Role modeling has been demonstrated as an effective strategy for such CCNS competencies as patient advocacy [5].

This skill of role modeling was put to the test while providing care to a 2-year-old Iraqi patient named "Marta." Marta suffered 45% full thickness burns to her lower back, buttocks, and both legs when an IED was thrown through the doorway of her home as her mother answered the door. Marta's mother and 2-month-old sister also were burned in the blast. They both made complete recoveries, but Marta had to stay in the ICU for extensive dressing changes and skin grafts. Unfortunately, her condition worsened, and she eventually was placed on the ventilator

Table 1
American Association of Critical-Care Nurses synergy model—patient characteristics

| Characteristic | Definition | Level of characteristic | Case study level |
|---|---|---|---|
| Complexity | Entanglement of two or more issues/systems (family, treatment therapy) | Level 1—highly complex (complex patient/family dynamics) Level 3—moderately complex Level 5—minimally complex (straightforward, routine) | Marta = 1 Hoda = 1 |
| Participation in decision making | Engagement of the patient/family in care decisions | Level 1—minimal participation (lack capacity/desire) Level 3—moderate participation Level 5—high participation (actively engaged, full involvement) | Marta = 1 Hoda = 5 |
| Participation in care | Engagement of the patient/family in aspects of care | Level 1—minimal participation (lack capacity/desire) Level 3—moderate participation Level 5—high participation (actively engaged, full involvement) | Marta = 1 Hoda = 3 |
| Predictability | Ability to expect a certain course of events/illness | Level 1—minimally predictable (uncertainty, rare) Level 3—moderately predictable Level 5—highly predictable (expected, common) | Marta = 1 Hoda = 1 |
| Resiliency | Ability to return to a prior level of functioning through the use of coping or compensatory mechanisms | Level 1—minimally resilient (brittle, low reserve capacity) Level 3—moderately resilient Level 5—highly resilient (possess endurance, high reserve capacity) | Marta = 1 Hoda = 1 |
| Resource availability | Extent to which resources are present in a situation (financial, psychological, social, and others) | Level 1—minimal resources (lack social/psychological support) Level 3—moderate resources Level 5—many resources (knowledgeable, strong social/psychological support) | Marta = 1 Hoda = 3 |
| Stability | Ability to maintain a state of equilibrium, responsiveness to therapy | Level 1—minimally stable (labile) Level 3—moderately stable Level 5—highly stable (constant) | Marta = 1 Hoda = 3 |
| Vulnerability | Extent of susceptibility to actual or potential stressors | Level 1—highly vulnerable (unprotected, fragile) Level 3—moderately vulnerable Level 5—minimally vulnerable (safe, able to protect against threats) | Marta = 1 Hoda = 3 |

*From* American Association of Critical-Care Nurses. The AACN synergy model for patient care. Available at: http://www.certcorp.org. Accessed April 30, 2007; with permission.

and unable to talk. Her family, especially her father, was at her bedside daily.

Unfortunately, because of an increased threat of a base attack corresponding to the upcoming Easter holiday, all hospital visitations for Iraqi patients were stopped. This was the first day Marta's father could not visit. Ventilated and unable to talk, Marta became restless with an increased heart rate, fever, and decreased blood pressure. As their eyes met, MAJ Freyling rubbed Marta's arm and softly told her it would be okay. Although Marta was not able to understand English, that touch crossed the language barrier and provided comfort in the absence of her father.

After a long period of unsuccessful attempts to treat her refractory hypotension and poor

Table 2
American Association of Critical-Care Nurses synergy model—nurse competencies

| Competency | Definition | Level of competency | Case study level |
|---|---|---|---|
| Advocacy and moral agency | Works on another's behalf; represents the concerns of patients and families; serves as a moral agent to resolve ethical and clinical issues | Level 1—works on behalf of patient, patient values congruent with own values<br>Level 3—works on behalf of patient and family, patient values may be different from own<br>Level 5—works on behalf of patient, family, and community; uses internal/external resources | Marta = 5<br>Hoda = 3 |
| Caring practices | Interventions and behaviors creating a therapeutic environment promoting comfort, healing, and compassion | Level 1—focuses on basic needs according to standards/protocols<br>Level 3—recognizes subtle changes in patient needs; attempts to tailor care to the patient<br>Level 5—interprets needs of patient and family; fully engaged | Marta = 5<br>Hoda = 5 |
| Clinical inquiry | Ongoing process of questioning and evaluating practice; incorporates research utilization and experiential learning | Level 1—follows current standards/guidelines; recognizes need for learning<br>Level 3—questions current policies/guidelines; compares/contrasts alternatives<br>Level 5—improves or individualizes policies/guidelines; performs literature review/research to make changes in current practice | Marta = 3<br>Hoda = 3 |
| Clinical judgment | Clinical reasoning used to deliver care, integrating knowledge and critical thinking to form clinical decisions | Level 1—collects and interprets basic data; adheres to protocols/algorithms<br>Level 3—collects and interprets complex data, comfortable deviating from protocols/algorithms when necessary<br>Level 5—collects and interprets multiple or conflicting data, anticipates problems based on past experience, delegates and collaborates with multidisciplinary team | Marta = 3<br>Hoda = 3 |

(*continued on next page*)

Table 2 (*continued*)

| Competency | Definition | Level of competency | Case study level |
|---|---|---|---|
| Collaboration | Working with the patient/ family and other members of the multidisciplinary team to promote optimal patient outcomes | Level 1—minimally collaborative, limited involvement of others<br>Level 3—moderately collaborative<br>Level 5—highly collaborative, all-inclusive | Marta = 3<br>Hoda = 5 |
| Facilitation in learning | Promotes learning for patients/families, staff, and the community both formally and informally; considers the educational level and the strengths or weaknesses of learners | Level 1—follows planned education strategies; learner is passive<br>Level 3—may incorporate varied teaching methods, considers the patient's needs<br>Level 5—develops educational plan with patient/family in collaboration with the multidisciplinary team; learner is active | Marta = 3<br>Hoda = 3 |
| Response to diversity | Ability to recognize, appreciate, and incorporate patient differences into the plan of care; recognizing the individuality of patients | Level 1—assesses diversity through a standard questionnaire, adheres to own belief system<br>Level 3—considers the individuality of the patient, inquires about differences<br>Level 5—actively responds to, anticipates, and integrates differences into the plan of care | Marta = 3<br>Hoda = 5 |
| Systems thinking | Ability to recognize the interconnected nature of a healthcare system, using a global perspective in clinical decision-making | Level 1—functions as the key resource for patients/ family, narrow view of resources<br>Level 3—moderate ability to recognize and react to patient/family needs as they move through a healthcare system, may use negotiation to obtain necessary resources<br>Level 5—holistic perspective, expertly navigates through the system effectively to ensure safe passage | Marta = 3<br>Hoda = 3 |

*From* American Association of Critical-Care Nurses. The AACN synergy model for patient care. Available at: http://www.certcorp.org. Accessed April 30, 2007; with permission.

ventilation and oxygenation, Marta died. Just as in the United States, advocating for family presence during end of life would have been part of the standard of patient care. The threat of a base attack, however, was too much of a risk for the base and for the family. Her family recognized that compassionate and caring practices were provided for Marta, especially when the staff intervened on her behalf with a long-standing cultural tradition. In Iraq, it is traditional to bury the dead within 24 hours [6]. The inability of her family to participate in care and decision making in Marta's final moments gave her nurse the opportunity to be her voice. Even though there was heightened security, the hospital staff made special arrangements for Marta's father and uncle to claim her body immediately so that they could uphold the tradition of burying her within 24 hours. Advocating for spiritual beliefs in the face of danger was the right thing to do to influence the sphere of care for this patient and her family.

## Diversity: snapshot of competency in a military ICU in Iraq

Response to diversity is a necessary nurse competency to achieve improved outcomes, especially for the Iraqi patient population. Being skilled at diversity means that an individual is able to recognize, appreciate, and incorporate differences into the provision of care [1,4]. In light of the significant cultural differences associated with the treatment of Arab women, mastering the competency of diversity was particularly important during this assignment in Iraq.

The most notable symbol of the status of Arab women is the covering of the hair in public with a veil that drapes around the head and neck and low on the forehead (and for some from the neck to the ankles) [6]. According to the Cultural Orientation Project, the root of the treatment of Arab women lies in the basic belief of a man's honor to family and the belief that men and women are unable or unwilling to control physical urges. It is also reported that Arab women are seen as dominated and repressed. Conversely, protection of women, by covering their bodies and not allowing them to make eye contact with other men, is seen by Arab women as evidence that they are loved and valued. Interestingly, some Arab women view Western freedoms as evidence of neglect and immorality [6].

Human rights abuse in Iraq was another cultural teaching of which MAJ Freyling became aware. Abuse in Iraq has been defined as torture, killings, disappearances, forced conscription, beatings, kidnappings, being held hostage, and ear amputations [7]. One study of 1991 households revealed that 82% of women had to obtain permission from a husband or male relative to access health care. Half of the men and women surveyed agreed there were reasons to restrict women's educational and employment opportunities and that a man had a right to beat his wife if

she did not obey him [7]. In addition, an Arab woman, whose family believes in honor killings, incurs the risk of death when damaging the family reputation by having sex with a man, dating a man, or even having her body seen by a man. This dishonor allows a male family member to murder the offending woman without repercussions [7]. This proved to be a major cultural concern in the care of a 17-year-old Arab female the authors will call "Hoda."

Hoda suffered a traumatic brain injury from an IED that was set off in front of her uncle's home in an effort to kill him. Shrapnel from the device entered Hoda's right frontal lobe and literally sliced through her brain, lodging in the occipital lobe. It was during her care that one could fully appreciate the synergistic relationship between linking the nurse competency of diversity and the patient characteristic of participation in care, and the engagement of the patient/family in aspects of care.

The nurses were told that Hoda was studying to be a teacher and that she came to the emergency room talking in English, despite the fact that brain matter was exposed. When MAJ Freyling began taking care of Hoda, it was postoperative day 1 for her. She had an intracranial pressure monitor, a ventriculostomy, ventilator support by means of an endotracheal tube, and was receiving sedation and analgesia intravenously. During rounds, the surgeons stated there was a good chance that Hoda would be killed once she returned home, as she did not have the customary male family member as an escort during her care to ensure she was not exposed to other males in the unit. Nurses began to make extra efforts to keep Hoda from exposure in the open bay area, as she was the only female in the ICU. They noticed that despite her sedation level, she often vigorously resisted any attempts at examining her abdomen and providing Foley catheter care. Enlisting the help of fellow nurses, a blanket wall was created around her bed while providing such care, and time was spent reassuring Hoda that she could not be seen by anyone. She kept her eyes closed most of the time.

Hoda's male cousin came to visit her on postoperative day 2. He cried when he saw her and expressed an emotional thank you to the nurses for caring for her. He said: "Put her in your heart the way I have put her in mine." MAJ Freyling assured him she would, and then she had the interpreter ask if there was anything special that should be done for Hoda. He said to keep her covered as much as possible and that her head should be covered when the rest of the family visited. MAJ Freyling told him she would ensure Hoda was covered, and that she would have a female nurse with her as much as possible. His responses led MAJ Freyling to believe that he was not so strict that he would recommend an honor killing for Hoda, but he may have had concerns about other family members. After weaning Hoda from the ventilator and having her begin to get up into a bedside chair, the ICU staff agreed to move her into another ICU, where, because of low census, they could wall off part of the ICU just for her. This gave Hoda privacy and took her away from the other male patients. Once she was ambulatory, Hoda began wearing her traditional veil while moving about the hospital with the physical therapist. Hoda's resiliency was amazing.

The CCNS is responsible for responding to diversity and ensuring patient and family needs are met, even when the needs are unusual to the health care staff [8]. In today's world, diversity exists in all areas. When working in a foreign land, however, response to diversity is a necessary nursing characteristic and key to improving patient outcomes. By applying the synergy model, MAJ Freyling was able to respond to the diversity of Hoda and her family by utilizing skills that included seeking information about her culture, working through the cultural differences, and tailoring the delivery of care to meet the diverse needs of her family.

## Summary

According to the synergy model, when patient characteristics and nurse competencies match, patient outcomes are optimized. The synergy model delineates three levels of outcomes: those derived from the patient, those derived from the nurse, and those derived from the health care system. A goal of nursing is to restore a patient to an optimal level of wellness as defined by patients and their families. The nurse characteristics can be considered competencies that are essential for those providing care to the critically ill. Whether applied in critical care settings in the United States or in Iraq, the synergy model provides an ideal framework to optimize positive outcomes for patients. The care of patients in Iraq can be complex and requires a competent skill set to help promote optimal outcomes. Both Marta and Hoda had conditions decreasing in stability and increasing in complexity (see Tables 1 and 2). At various points, both were no longer predictable in their continuum of care; resiliency was questionable, and vulnerability was high. Hoda had family support to help guide the decisions being made in her care; however, Marta was dependent on United States military health care providers to guide her plan of care at the end of life. In caring for these two challenging patients, MAJ Freyling was able to utilize all eight nursing competencies to reflect an integration of her knowledge, skills, and experience. The synergy model provided her with a framework upon which to base her practice.

## Acknowledgements

The opportunity to complete course requirements to be eligible for the CCNS examination was made possible by Carol Hartigan, RN, MSN, Director of the AACN Certification Corporation, the AACN Scholarship Fund, and faculty at the Acute and Critical Care Clinical Nurse Specialist Program at Georgetown University School of Nursing & Health Studies.

## References

[1] American Association of Critical-Care Nurses. The AACN synergy model for patient care. Available at: http://www.certcorp.org. Accessed April 30, 2007.

[2] Cohen S, Crego N, Cuming R, et al. The synergy model and the role of clinical nurse specialists in a multihospital system. Am J Crit Care 2002;11(5): 436–46.

[3] Curley MAQ. Patient–nurse synergy: optimizing patients' outcomes. Am J Crit Care 1998;7:64–72.

[4] Hardin SR, Kaplow R. Synergy for clinical excellence: the AACN synergy model for patient care. Boston: Jones and Bartlett; 2005.

[5] Von Rueden KT, Hartsock RL. Nursing practice through the cycle of trauma. In: McQuillan KA, Von Rueden KT, Hartsock RL, et al, editors. Trauma nursing: from resuscitation to rehabilitation. 3rd edition. Philadelphia: Saunders; 2002. p. 108–28.

[6] The Cultural Orientation Project. Iraqis—their history and culture. Refugee fact sheet no. 11. 2004. Available at: http://www.culturalorientation.net/iraqi/ilife.html. Accessed April 30, 2007.

[7] Adams M. 2004. Human rights abuse in Iraq. Women & Infants' Hospital of Rhode Island. Available at: http://www.womenandinfants.com/body.cfm?id=388&;chunkiid=75563. Accessed April 30, 2007.

[8] Hardin SR. In response to diversity. In: Hardin SR, Kaplow R, editors. Synergy for clinical excellence. Synergy model for patient care. Boston: Jones and Bartlett; 2005. p. 91–7.

ELSEVIER
SAUNDERS

Crit Care Nurs Clin N Am 20 (2008) 31–40

CRITICAL CARE
NURSING CLINICS
OF NORTH AMERICA

# Stateside Care of Marines and Sailors Injured in Iraq at the National Naval Medical Center in Bethesda, Maryland

Loretta J. Aiken, RN, MSN*,
Patrice Bibeau, RN, MSN, CCRN, CDR, NC, USN,
Barbie Cilento, RN, M Ed, MSN,
Eddie Lopez, RN, MSN, LCDR, NC, USN

*National Naval Medical Center, 8901 Wisconsin Avenue, Bethesda, MD 20889-5600, USA*

The National Naval Medical Center (NNMC) is located in Bethesda, Maryland, just outside of Washington, DC. It is often referred to simply as "the Naval Hospital" and is considered by the US Navy to be the flagship of navy medicine [1]. This world-renowned teaching hospital complex has provided care to war heroes serving in the United States military for more than 65 years. It is also referred to as "the President's Hospital," whose mission is to assure the readiness and care of the uniformed services and their families [1].

Before the start of the current conflict, it had been several years since the United States was involved in major combat operations. As a result, health care providers had limited experience in treating traumatic injuries associated with war fighting and the sequelae of infection and sepsis. Early lessons were learned in 2003 aboard the United States Naval Ship Comfort Tanker–Auxiliary Hospital 20 while treating primarily Iraqi soldiers, civilians, and some members of the coalition forces [2]. For the first time, many of the ICU team members were exposed to patients

who had gunshot wounds, traumatic amputations, open and closed head injuries, blunt and penetrating blast injuries, burns covering a large body surface area, acute respiratory distress syndrome, and sepsis. Those experiences helped refine the approach taken to care for the service members and civilians who are critically injured and arrive at NNMC by way of the US Air Force Medical Evacuation (MEDEVAC) system.

More than 1600 casualties have been admitted to NNMC from Operation IRAQI FREEDOM/ Operation ENDURING FREEDOM (OIF/OEF) [3]. Not all the casualties have been admitted to the critical care department; however, those requiring comprehensive multidisciplinary medical care are admitted to the ICU. The injuries sustained have been severe, often changing lives forever. Many of the wounded have survived, whereas a few have not. Whatever the outcome, the health care team has continuously provided state-of-the art trauma support to the wounded, and psychosocial support to the patient and his/her family. Additionally, "care for the caregiver" assistance is available for the multidisciplinary team, whether provided formally, through counseling services available from Psychiatry or Pastoral Services, or informally, through the verbalization of their experiences with colleagues, family members, or friends. In either instance, nurses use various means to cope successfully with the multisystem, trauma patient population from OIF/OEF.

The views expressed in this article are those of the authors and do not reflect the official policy of the Department of the Navy, the Department of Defense, or the US Government.

* Corresponding author.

*E-mail address:* Loretta.Aiken@med.navy.mil (L.J. Aiken).

The ICU nursing staff has encountered several casualties, evoking various emotions in response to the devastating injuries sustained by the wounded service members. The resilience of the health care team is evident in their daily interactions as they consistently maintain professional composure while providing compassionate, patient-centered care despite the inherent challenges. Some nurses and other members of the trauma team have spouses, brothers, and friends serving in Iraq, which makes them even more dedicated to providing the best nursing care to the wounded warriors.

MEDEVAC admissions are intense times and require the nurse to put aside his/her emotions to provide the best care possible. The entire nursing staff demonstrates tireless skill and expertise while providing demanding physical nursing care and addressing the psychosocial needs of the patients and their families. Such nursing care is truly an art.

The reception of these casualties has become systematic and refined to a science. The team's response depends on the number of casualties and the types of injuries they have sustained. Information about an incoming wounded warrior is relayed by the MEDEVAC office in the form of the patient movement report. This report contains a brief history of the mechanism of injury, the procedures, medication, and therapies, and the patient's condition. The patient movement report can be available from days to hours before the patient's arrival and it is what directs the team's action and initial plan of treatment. One to three Critical Care Aeromedical Transport (CCAT) casualties are expected on most MEDEVAC flights, but there can be more. To date, the highest number of CCAT casualties received for one mission has been seven. The medical center is able to admit and care for this high number of casualties safely and expeditiously because of the streamlined admission process.

**First hours**

When the wounded arrive at NNMC, a well-orchestrated team approach is implemented to meet the patients' needs and promote the best possible outcomes. Wounded service members are initially admitted to the Trauma Service, whose members consult with various subspecialties, allied health professionals, and administrative staff. A collaborative approach is used by the team to develop an individualized plan of care. An ideal ICU admission team is composed of three staff members, including a minimum of one registered nurse (RN) and two hospital corpsmen, which is the navy title given to enlisted personnel assigned to the medical occupational specialty that provides patient care under the supervision of licensed medical providers; other branches of the armed services refer to them as medics. A respiratory therapist must be nearby to manage intubated patients and those demonstrating respiratory difficulties. Also, the administrative staff is equally important, to assist with telephone communications, transport laboratory specimens, and support family members and other visitors.

Newly arriving patients can require 1:1 or 2:1 nursing care for extended periods of time because of the severity of the injuries, hemodynamic instability, or labor-intensive diagnostic procedures; therefore, adequate staffing is crucial. The MEDEVAC aircraft usually arrives in the evening from the US Army's Landstuhl Regional Medical Center (LRMC) in Germany. The patients are then transported from nearby Andrews Air Force Base, Maryland, to NNMC by ground ambulance, arriving in the ICU approximately 1 hour later. The evening arrival time occurs around the change of shift, which provides maximum support because personnel from both the day and night shifts are present. The day shift staff is sometimes asked to stay late and the in-coming shift is called and asked to come in early. Some staff members who are not scheduled to work may be asked to come in for a 4- to 6-hour period. In these situations, the nursing staff eagerly volunteers.

The day shift charge nurse plans room assignments for each patient by considering the acuity and monitoring equipment that will be required. Once rooms are assigned, the corpsmen start to prepare for the admission. The rooms are stocked with a limited amount of supplies and equipment to minimize waste and decrease the likelihood of cross-contamination. A set of documents is stamped with the patient's data using a preadmission addressograph card to ensure accuracy and completeness. Isolation carts, culture bottles, culture swabs, and biowaste containers are available in each room.

The ICU is divided into two identical ten-bed sections (pods), with five rooms on each side of a hallway. Large fire-safety doors separate these units. Because of the prevalence of *Acinetobacter baumannii* in the soil of Iraq, whenever possible, patients are admitted into only one of the 10-bed pods of the ICU to keep one unit as an isolation unit and the other as a "clean" unit. All patients from Iraq are considered contaminated with *Acinetobacter baumannii*, which could compromise other patients. Therefore, on arrival, the injured are immediately placed on contact and droplet precautions.

As the casualties come into the ICU, the Air Force medical personnel caring for each patient are directed to the specified room. Patients arrive minutes apart in a span of a half hour and are in various medical conditions, from stable to extremely critical. The charge nurse, nursing supervisor, and medical support assistant page the physicians and facilitate the administrative admission process. For each patient, the scenario is similar: the primary RN receives a report from the Air Force medical personnel and performs a quick visual assessment of the patient. The patient movement report information specifies ventilator settings, intravenous fluids, and medications for the transition from the transport equipment to the bedside devices. The patient is quickly removed from the litter, placed into the ICU bed, and connected to the monitors. While some ICU staff members acquire a set of specimen samples and cultures to include blood, sputum, skin, urine, and wound, another staff member begins to expose the patient by removing dressings and bandages so that the providers can perform thorough assessments related to their specialty. The physician teams focus on the immediate treatment of the patient and write the orders for each individual intervention based on the type of injuries seen. The nursing staff then activates the orders.

In the ICU admission process, the nurse begins the patient's reorientation immediately by introducing himself/herself. At this point, the nurse tells the patient where he/she is. At the same time, the first part of the nursing assessment is started. Observations are noted and documented as to the patient's physical and psychologic status, which can be a very emotional time for the nurse because he/she is viewing the young person and inspecting the debilitating injuries that can become fatal or life altering. Some of these patients are not much younger than the nurses taking care of them and some of the nurses have siblings that are the same age as some of the injured. It is also especially hard for the corpsmen, because they are even younger than some of the nurses and more likely to be the same age as the wounded warrior (Figs. 1 and 2).

## ICU course

Depending on the patient's injuries, the next few hours can be extremely busy. For traumatic brain injury patients, trips to CT scan occur as soon as possible. These trips require the ICU RN, a respiratory therapist, a physician, and a corpsman to accompany the patient off the unit for 45 to 60 minutes. For those with extremity fractures or joint injuries, multiple radiographs are performed at the bedside. Some warriors require 10 to 20 films each. After completion of the initial assessment, immediate procedures or surgery may be required. As a result, the ICU team may need to transport the patient to multiple departments at a moment's notice.

Nurses provide the minute-to-minute, hands-on care and observation that is vital to the patient. During the first few hours that the injured warrior is stateside, the nurse–patient–family bonds are formed. Families are pivotal in the recovery process and are encouraged to interact with their loved ones. One way to try to elicit responses from the patient is to bring the family members into the room as soon as possible. They are informed of the patient's condition and status, and they learn what to expect when seeing their son or daughter for the first time. For some, this step is really difficult. All the worry, fear, and extreme emotional distress can be a big shock when they see their loved one in such a compromised state. In all scenarios, the nurse is the primary support and provides a shoulder to cry on when needed.

After the reality of the situation sets in, the family members demonstrate various responses to the injury of their loved one, including grief, anger, and denial. They know their loved one is ill and may not make it through this critical time. From the onset, the nursing staff plays a fundamental role in assisting family members with their emotional responses. Visiting hours are open (24/7) to allow family members the time needed to begin to deal with the situation at hand. An open dialog is also instrumental to a successful recovery, and so the nurses keep the families abreast of new developments in the patient's care. As a result, it is common for family members to consider the nurse as their contact for all medical information regarding the patient.

Because the RNs work 12-hour shifts three or four times a week, nurses are the constant focal point for the family and share the emotional experiences they have to endure. The patient and family are considered to be one family unit and care is directed to keep them all informed. Nurses sometimes joke about the "mini medical school education" they provide. The families become very involved with every single aspect of the care

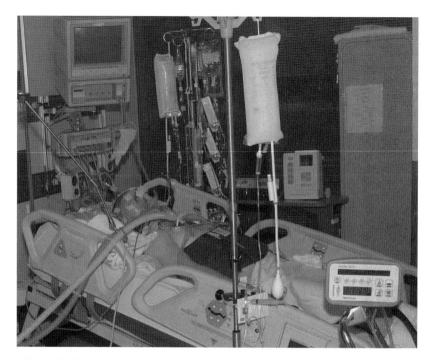

Fig. 1. Multisystem trauma ICU patient with traumatic brain injury from OIF conflict.

and can readily quote laboratory values, radio-graph results, temperatures, surgeries, antibiotic levels, and culture results.

Many times, the families become attached to a particular nurse and may become distant with other nurses during that individual's day off. It is not uncommon for this nurse to experience feelings of guilt on leaving at the end of the shift because of the bond that has been formed. Some family members become wary of other nurses who are unfamiliar to them. As a result, the nurse and the family learn to deal with the complexity of the patient's injuries and have to work through their own profound feelings of anxiety and fear of what might happen during days away from the partic-ular patient. Consequently, it is not at all un-common for nurses and family member to stay in contact for years after the relationship develops in the ICU.

## Injuries of the war wounded in critical care

The OIF/OEF conflict has lasted 4 years, and there have been peaks and valleys in the number of wounded arriving each month. The staff at NNMC constantly learns from these war experi-ences and they make improvements in the management of trauma from battle injuries and other injuries associated with military duty. Mil-itary medicine has broken new ground in the treatment of head injuries, blast injuries, fracture care, infectious disease management, and pain management.

Blast injuries are by far the signature injury of the Iraq War and can cause multiple levels of trauma. For example, a humvee may be hit by a round of mortar fire that propels the vehicle many feet into the air. Projectiles, clouds of bacteria-laced debris, and fire can cause the troops to be maimed. Shell shock can be generated from a blast wave of high pressure spreading 1600 feet per second [4], which results in an acceleration-deceleration injury to the brain [5]. The movement of the brain matter inside the skull causes bruising at multiple sites, edema, and pressure, and possi-ble bleeding within the closed vault. The occu-pants not only suffer blast injuries but also major impact injuries because of the sequences of events. Added to that scenario, the service member might be rescued from the vehicle and then be subjected to the additional trauma of gun-shot wounds from sniper fire.

Battle wounds can be sustained from many different mechanisms, but the most devastating injuries by far are those resulting from the

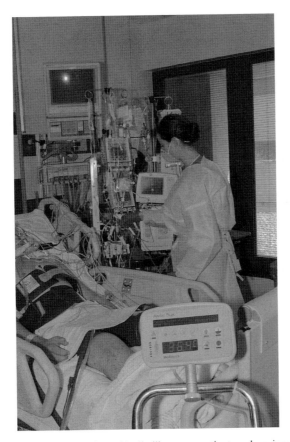

Fig. 2. ICU RN assessing critically ill trauma patient, and equipment.

improvised explosive devices (IEDs). Some of the service members experience traumatic brain injury, without visible wounds, just by being in close proximity to repeated explosions. The constant barrage of blast noise generates waves of sound that can rupture eardrums and cause brain injuries. The noise can be caused by grenades, missiles, IEDs, mortar rounds, or the gun shot sounds of fire fights and snipers. Service members have coined the phrase, "having my bell rung," when they discuss their traumatic brain injuries from blast explosions.

Severely head-injured patients come to NNMC and present with their own set of challenges. Their neurologic status is difficult to assess because of heavy sedation during the flight, and the extent of head injury is not well known until the massive swelling of the brain subsides. Neurologic care of the traumatic brain injury patient has shown remarkable advances since the beginning of the war. At local field hospitals in Iraq, neurosurgeons perform surgery immediately to reduce the

extent of swelling of the brain (eg, a procedure known as "craniectomy" surgically removes part of the skull, allowing the brain to expand).

The nursing care for these patients may necessitate bedside intracranial monitoring and brain oxygen tissue and brain perfusion monitoring, in addition to keeping track of everything else a severe critical care patient needs. Adding all that to the many trips to CT scan, Angiography, MRI, and the operating room, the person-hours and staff effort is astonishing, keeping in mind that these new technologies require RNs to possess advanced knowledge of these types of interventions. Sometimes, the nurse may have no idea if the patient is able to comprehend what is being said but will repeatedly tell the patient that he/she is back in the United States at NNMC.

Pain relief is of utmost importance to adequate care of the wounded. Because of the nature and severity of war injuries, major advances have been made in pain management. By using local blocks, intravenous narcotics, sedation, infusion catheters (eg, patient-controlled analgesia and epidurals), low-dose ketamine infusions, oral methadone, and topical narcotic patches, great strides have been made in the way pain is controlled. Pain medication balls or similar devices are commonly used to bathe wounds with a continual wash of local anesthetic to dull the acuteness of pain. New technology has been implemented and is constantly updated to ensure everything possible is being done to alleviate pain.

Because of the large numbers of blast injuries that result in bone, muscle, and tissue loss, knowledge has been gained in the way we manage amputation injuries. To be classified as an amputation, the whole hand, arm, foot, or leg must be totally gone. Digits do not count as amputations. Body armor can protect the torso, but limbs are highly susceptible to devastating trauma from blasts. Bereavement and coping are two major issues war fighters face with all amputation injuries. Some can end up in severe emotional turmoil because of their loss, and many disciplines interact with patients and families to help with their acceptance of their injuries.

Traumatic brain injury service members require frequent reorientation and the staff has to remind them repeatedly that they are safe and back in the United States. Many have no recollection of their injury or even their MEDEVAC flight. The last thing they might remember is the heat of battle. Their next cognitive moment may be days or weeks later and several thousand miles from the battlefield. The staff caring for the war wounded tells them what has happened and keeps them informed of what is being done for them. In just about every case, medical personnel and commands from the field in Iraq will call to check on these servicemen and women. The injured may never realize that, all along the long route home, possibly hundreds of people have worked with precision and dedication to get them back to NNMC. The Air Force transport team even leaves them a small guardian angel pin and a note about the transport back to the United State. These pins are a way for the flight staff to communicate to those they watched over during the flight.

Many warriors are unaware of the extent of their injuries until they are awakened at NNMC. Most of them have been intubated and sedated from the time of their injury in the battlefield up until they are safe in the ICU setting. When he/she is awake enough for ventilator weaning, the wounded warrior is apprised of the battle wounds by the medical staff. The health care team is always sensitive in relaying this type of information because it can be devastating to the service member. Family and nursing support is essential at this time, and many times, pastoral support is used to assist the patient and family with the emotional response to the altered body image.

## Services provided to the patient and family

Marine and navy officials notify family members of the patient's injury as soon as possible. Sometimes, in cases of severe injuries, a family member will fly directly to Germany and accompany the transport flight back home. Up to three family members may have transportation from their homes paid for by the Service. The liaisons make accommodations either on the base or as close to the base as possible. They provide transportation for the family members to and from the hospital. The base has two Fisher Houses (which are analogous to the Ronald McDonald houses in the civilian sector), a navy lodge (motel), and two barracks to house families. On occasion, family members arrive before the wounded warrior does and are sometimes waiting in the hallway to give words of love and comfort as the patient first arrives in the ICU.

Because of the number of wounded who have been at NNMC, we have learned that for the patient to recover, the family also needs to be cared for. The entire staff at NNMC makes every effort to help the families in crisis. Some family members need more help than others, and the army, navy, or marine liaison and social workers help with referrals to the Navy Marine Relief Society. This society assists with all types of loans, bill payments, transportation, and other needed services. Sometimes the family is even given temporary use of a vehicle, which is donated for family members' use during their long stays at the hospital center.

The social work and case management departments at NNMC are vital in the recovery process. The social worker, discharge planner, and case manager develop a comprehensive plan that includes integrating each health care discipline's recommendations into the overall discharge plan. These disciplines assist with allocation of resources to carry out the plan and help with the appropriate referrals and necessary consultations. They also meet with family members to help with logistics related to food, lodging, pre-existing family conflicts, and the impact of the injured warrior's condition on the various family members.

When a wounded service member arrives at NNMC, he/she receives a quilt that has been made by one of the chapters of the Quilts for Valor organization [6]. Attached to each quilt is the name and hometown of the maker, and a personal note to the wounded warrior who is receiving it. These quilts are just one example of the many dedicated individuals throughout the country who support the troops.

A well-known athletic shoe company provides each wounded warrior a voucher for one pair of new shoes. One organization donates backpacks that contain personal care items such as toiletries, shaving gear, nail clippers, music CDs, books, gum, bar candy, and snacks. All returning injured servicemen are given a gift certificate to purchase uniforms or personal clothing items. Often, wounded warriors are given pillows, CD players, or other small electronic devices, not to mention the personal gifts from music performers or Hollywood personalities. Video movies, movie passes, autographs, photographs, and memorabilia are handed out by visiting celebrities. Holiday meals, family parties, and gala special events have been planned, catered, and served by large hotels and local food establishments. Churches have donated food, clothing, and all sorts of items for patients and family members. Beauty shops supply complimentary gift certificates for wives and mothers, and hotels often provide free accommodations for families of war wounded. The contributions are far too many to mention, but all efforts from the various support groups are appreciated by families and service members.

Family members often refer to the stays at NNMC as the "perpetual crisis state" because the road is always bumpy and uncertain, so NNMC attempts to reduce the stress with various activity diversions for the families. NNMC has an avenue of shops on the first floor by the main cafeteria that families frequent. Although not quite a shopping mall, it allows them to browse boutique items from street venders, go to the Navy Federal Credit Union to conduct financial business, check out books from the base library, or even visit the barber shop or uniform store. The Navy Federal Credit Union will send bedside representatives to discuss financial matters with wounded warriors and their families. Café Leisure is a recreational service used to help break the monotony for family members being away from their homes.

The café offers some type of entertainment that may include a movie and a dinner. Many movies are available throughout the hospital to help families pass a little time away from the bedside.

## Examples of ICU care

It is 0800 on Friday morning and the ICU charge nurse has been notified to expect two MEDEVAC admissions around 1700 in the evening. Both of the admissions are war wounded with injuries from an IED blast. Marine #1 is a 22-year-old who sustained injuries to the head resulting in a subdural hematoma, traumatic amputation of the left leg, and large open wounds to the abdomen and right arm. His left femoral artery was exposed on the battlefield and an immediate tourniquet was applied above the amputation. He was alert at the time of injury but soon lost consciousness when transported to the field hospital. At the field hospital, Marine #1 was assessed and a determination was made to transfer him immediately to LRMC for further treatment. He suffered a cardiac arrest while being transported to Germany but had a return of spontaneous circulation 2 minutes after cardiopulmonary resuscitation effort began. He was placed on a ventilator and vasoactive support started in flight. Because of his blood volume loss, he received a large volume of crystalloids and colloids. Marine #1 was stabilized in Germany, and the neurosurgeon performed a cranioplasty for his head injury. The traumatic amputated left leg needed immediate surgical revision, and the open wounds in the abdomen and right arm were cleaned, irrigated, and drained. Marine #1 is transported to NNMC where he will continue to receive treatment in the ICU.

Marine #2 is a 20-year-old who sustained injuries in an IED blast to his face, eyes, right arm, and abdomen. He has been conscious since the blast. He is unable to see because his left eye was enucleated, and scrap metal is embedded in the right eye and the right side of his face. His abdomen sustained a large wound, where his spleen and part of his liver were removed. He has lost a large volume of blood during the actual injury and successive surgeries. He has been transfused a total of 24 units of blood products and he continues to ooze bloody drainage from his abdomen. He has a large wound on his right forearm that was closed in the field hospital, but he developed compartment syndrome in the right arm, which has since compromised circulation to the lower part of his right arm. He has been on hourly circulation checks since the hematoma was drained and vascular surgery was performed on the arm in Germany. He is being transported to NNMC's ICU for monitoring of his neurologic and bleeding status.

As both marines entered the ICU, their families were anxiously waiting to see them. The staff of NNMC let the families into the room. It was an emotional time to watch moms, dads, spouses, and siblings plead with their loved one to get better. They survived the ICU course with their families and the staff at the bedside encouraging them each day. They were eventually transferred from the ICU to a poly-trauma Veterans Administration medical facility.

**Emotional aspects of care**

The ICU staff must be aware of their emotions throughout the patient's ICU course. Emotion is defined as "an affective state of consciousness in which joy, sorrow, fear, hate, or the like is experienced" [7]. Emotions can run high for the patient and family and the nursing staff at any time and consequently, awareness is the key to ensuring the provision of quality care.

The emotional preparation for a patient's arrival is not officially discussed because it is assumed to be part of the job. Many nurses focus on the medical care requirements, commenting on the need for such items as a mechanical ventilator, an intracranial pressure monitor, a neurologic tissue oxygenation monitor, or a basic hemodynamic monitoring system. Obtaining these items is the first step in preparing for the patient's admission, ensuring a smooth transition from the flight line in Germany to the United States. When the room is totally prepared with all these items in order, the staff is then able to ponder the injuries that each patient has sustained. They will discuss the impending admission and strategize a care plan with the multidisciplinary team. Others prepare for admissions by reflecting on the patients they cared for previously and will adapt lessons learned to the current scenario. Their response may not be uniform, but in either instance, a mental preparation occurs to ensure that the patient is admitted, stabilized, and started on the road to recovery. Nurses have learned to use various mechanisms to cope successfully with the multisystem, trauma patient population from OIF/OEF.

One example of such resilience was displayed in the care of a 22-year-old marine who acquired a devastating head injury from shrapnel that pierced his skull during hand-to-hand contact with an insurgent. It was later learned that this young man had jumped on a grenade to protect several members of his platoon, using his Kevlar helmet and body to protect others from the effects of the blast. His heroic efforts were recognized 2 years later by his being the first marine to receive the Medal of Honor since 1970 [8].

This heroic marine was transferred from LRMC by CCAT. His neurologic injuries were identified as devastating at LRMC, yet his parents requested that he be transferred to NNMC for further evaluation. The multidisciplinary team was prepared for his arrival, having received a report from LRMC and the MEDEVAC coordinator. The Trauma Service and Neurosurgery team were quick to evaluate and discuss treatment options with his parents while supporting them as they lovingly stood by their son's bedside. Despite their best efforts, the patient's injuries were too severe and, consequently, he passed away shortly thereafter. All members of the health care team felt the tragic loss of this individual's life. Those directly involved with this marine's care spent additional time with the family, encouraging them to reminisce about his childhood and love of the Marine Corps. Others provided support to the direct care givers, assisting them with performing postmortem care, completing miscellaneous documents, and providing care to their other patients. Many discussed the death quietly among themselves, acknowledging the harsh realities of war, as a means to cope with the situation at hand. In the end, the staff felt some comfort in knowing that they did all that they could to assist the patient and his family during this difficult time.

Another example involved a marine in his early twenties who succumbed to severe abdominal and orthopedic injuries. Having been in the ICU for approximately 1 week, the staff established a relationship with the family, particularly the patient's mother, wife, and young daughter. When his death occurred, it was particularly difficult because the family was not ready to let go and became quite distraught with his passing. To deal effectively with this situation, the staff required the support of the psychiatrist and chaplain on duty to assist with the wife's distressed reaction and their own response to the gravity of the situation. Periodic sessions were then established with the Psychiatry Service to assist the health care team in dealing with the emotions they encountered while caring for these individuals and their family members. These sessions were found to be especially helpful in the early months of OIF/OEF, particularly with the increase in the numbers of casualties. Eventually, the sessions were not needed on a routine basis, although individual counseling is encouraged for anyone who needs support.

## Joys of recovery

Despite the numerous experiences with death and loss, stories also exist of medical recovery and successful healing. One courageous marine sustained injury to both upper extremities, requiring two amputations, one above the elbow and another below the elbow. The courage and consistently optimistic attitude displayed by this individual, and his parents who were both health care professionals, was truly admirable. He eventually transferred from the ICU to the surgical ward and was later discharged. He apparently returned to stateside duty, and reportedly was seen at a televised patriotic concert, proudly saluting during the ceremony honoring service members for their contributions during OIF/OEF. His recovery and eventual return to the workforce were an affirmation of the quality care provided by the health care team, enabling these brave men and women who have served our country the opportunity to live life as they so choose. The health care team is proud to be part of these individuals' recoveries.

Another example involved the care of a reporter who sustained severe closed head injuries. Having been treated at NNMC for more than 30 days, many of the health care team established a close rapport with this patient, his wife, children, and siblings. His room was decorated with photographs of family and friends, offering a snapshot of his love of life while facilitating the dialog of caregivers with the patient and his family. He was eventually stabilized and then transferred to a rehabilitation facility for further treatment. The staff learned later that the patient and his family wanted to return to produce a story on what he had experienced, showcasing his care and those who were instrumental in his recovery. Many were touched by these actions and the televised report that ensued. The joy of this patient's recovery was evident on everyone's faces as they greeted the family at NNMC and during the televised report. The staff was proud that the job they perform on a daily basis received this recognition by one patient on national television. Such recognition undoubtedly provided a boost to the health care team's morale, rejuvenating their ability to continue to do the job that they perform so well.

The nursing staff frequently receives pictures and letters from patients or their families. Often, patients and family members visit the unit after recuperating from their injuries. These visits are very special and meaningful for the staff, providing a feeling of extreme accomplishment. The staff will talk about it for days and will make sure that everyone knows how this service member is doing. A bulletin board in the ICU has notes tacked up on it. Every day, one finds the staff members eating lunch and reading all the notes on the board. At times, one hears, "I can't believe how well he is doing." The sense of pride in a job well done resounds throughout the ICU.

## Summary

The emotions that an ICU health care provider experiences on a daily basis can certainly vary, depending on the outcomes of the patients served. Each individual may cope with these emotionally straining patient care scenarios in a personal and unique manner; however, they do find the courage and strength to provide the quality care required with the utmost professionalism and dedication. Caring for this patient population is awe inspiring and fulfills this special health care team's patriotic duty to serve their country during this time of war.

Every single member of the entire health team at NNMC is important in helping the service member and family cope with, and deal with, the anguish of sustained injuries and the need for extensive hospital stays. From the kitchen and nutrition staff, to the housekeeping and maintenance staff, to the professional and nonprofessional divisions, the unwavering commitment from the entire command is incredible. Family members will often write to NNMC about acts of kindness they have received and the letters will be filled with amazement about how so many people, from so many different departments, interacted with them in a memorable way during such a stressful time in their lives.

## Acknowledgment

The authors would like to give a special thank you to Susan Dionne, RN, MSN, CAPT, NC, USN for her support in this project.

## References

[1] NNMC homepage. Available at: http://www.bethesda. med.navy.mil/Visitor/About_Us/. Accessed April 1, 2007.

[2] USNS Comfort (T-AH 20). Available at: http://www. comfort.navy.mil/history.html. Accessed April 1, 2007.

[3] NNMC Casualty Affairs Database. Retrieved March 4, 2007 from NNMC restricted share drive.

[4] Glasser R. A shock waveof brain injuries. The Washington Post April 8, 2007; p. B1, B5.

[5] Hickey JV. The clinical practice of neurological and neurosurgical nursing. 5th edition. Philadelphia: Lippincott Williams & Wilkins; 2003.

[6] Quilts for valor. 2006. Available at: http://www. houseofhanson.com/qov.html. Accessed April 21, 2007.

[7] Dictionary.com. 2007. Available at: http://www.dic tionary.com. Accessed: April 16, 2007.

[8] Fuentes G. Posthumous honor: corporal's medal of honor is first for marine since Vietnam. Navy Times November 27, 2006;20.

ELSEVIER
SAUNDERS

CRITICAL CARE
NURSING CLINICS
OF NORTH AMERICA

Crit Care Nurs Clin N Am 20 (2008) 41–49

# Critical Care Nurses' Experiences Caring for the Casualties of War Evacuated from the Front Line: Lessons Learned and Needs Identified

Deborah J. Kenny, RN, PhD, LTC, AN, USA[a,*],
Mary S. Hull, RN, MSN, APN, LTC, AN, USA[b]

[a]Uniformed Services University of the Health Sciences, 4301 Jones Bridge Road, Bethesda, MD 20814, USA
[b]Inpatient Psychiatry, Landstuhl Regional Medical Center, CMR 402, Box 959,
APO AE 09180, Landstuhl, Germany

People will always be the lifeblood of a healthcare organization. They must be cared for and nurtured for the organization to grow and prosper in these rapidly changing times...... The toll of unmanaged stress and the effects of compassion fatigue leave a mark. Alcohol and drug abuse, divorce and broken relationships, anxiety, depression, professional dysfunction, errors, cynicism, or loss of compassion are each part of the human endeavor that pushes human limits [1].

Caring for critically ill patients can be stressful. Some literature suggests that it is more pronounced than the stress associated with caring for patients who are not in an ICU [2]. However, many studies have reported differences in stress levels between ICU nurses and those working in non-ICU areas. Older studies comparing these stress levels found no differences related to the work environment [3,4]. More recent studies have begun investigating relationships between different work factors and stress levels among ICU and non-ICU nurses. One study reported that although ICU nurses reported higher uncertainty, work complexity, and higher decision

authority, they also experienced lower emotional exhaustion than non-ICU nurses [5]. Other recent articles examined moral distress of ICU nurses as it relates to futile care and other ethical issues arising from caring for critically ill patients, such as helplessness, unrecognized grief, and emotional exhaustion [6–9]. In addition, higher anxiety experienced by ICU nurses was associated with poorer performance on tasks [10]. The provision of what ICU nurses believed to be *care not resulting in benefit* caused the highest levels of stress, which unfavorably affected job satisfaction and retention [11]. It also adversely affected the overall well-being of nurses. Regardless of study results, the literature supports the fact that caring for patients in an ICU environment results in nurse stress, which impacts both patients and nurses.

This article examines the stressors of nurses working in the ICUs of two U.S. military medical treatment facilities (MTFs) before and after the beginning of the wars in Iraq (*Operation Iraqi Freedom* [OIF]) and Afghanistan (*Operation Enduring Freedom* [OEF]). The MTF in Europe is a stabilization and evacuation point for ill and wounded United States soldiers. The second MTF, in the United States, is where wounded soldiers arrive from overseas for definitive care. During peacetime, the mission of both MTFs is to care for active duty, retired, and family member beneficiaries. In addition to identified stressors of ICU nurses, background discussion of the concepts of secondary traumatization and compassion fatigue is presented. Coping mechanisms

The views expressed in this article are those of the authors and do not reflect the official policy of the Department of the Army, the Department of Defense, or the United States Government.

* Corresponding author.
*E-mail address:* deb.kenny@us.army.mil
(D.J. Kenny).

0899-5885/08/$ - see front matter. Published by Elsevier Inc.
doi:10.1016/j.ccell.2007.10.013

described by the ICU nurses in both environments are illustrated. Lastly, solutions and suggestions for alleviating stress, potential burnout, or compassion fatigue are offered.

## Method for collecting data

A large number of soldiers injured in OIF and OEF arriving from the war zone to fixed MTFs (as opposed to the transportable, temporary nature of a combat support hospital) for definitive treatment are first cared for by ICU nurses. The authors wanted to compare stressors and coping mechanisms of these nurses both before and after the beginning of the wars. A simple, long-answer questionnaire was developed by the authors to examine the variables of interest (Fig. 1). After obtaining approval from the Institutional Review Boards (IRBs) at both MTFs, the questionnaire was distributed to active duty, reserve, and civilian nurses who worked in the ICUs at both facilities. The questionnaire was accompanied by a cover letter stating that participation was voluntary, and participants were asked not to put their names on the questionnaires. Completed questionnaires were to be placed in an envelope located at the nursing station and were collected

by the authors 1 week after distribution. Another check was made 2 weeks after distribution for any other questionnaires that might have been completed. The envelopes were then removed from the units and the questionnaires given a number. Fifty questionnaires were distributed at the MTF in the United States and 50 in Europe. Nine completed questionnaires were returned from the U.S. MTF and nine from Europe, yielding a response rate of 18%. The low response rate of the nurses is typical at both MTFs and may reflect many factors, including the amount of research occurring at the facilities, the workload of the nurses, and the increased stress of the environment. Although the authors and editors recognize that 18% is a low response rate, they believe that the anecdotal information provided by these participants should be shared because it offers a glimpse at how nurses on these front lines perceive their situation and how they respond to increased stressors and workload. This information affords a possible starting point for additional studies on this area of nursing and patient care. The responses were collated, analyzed for content, and used to illustrate stressors as described by the nurses themselves within the typical ICU environment of both MTFs before

---

**"Stressors and Coping Mechanisms of ICU Nurses Before and After OIF/OEF"**
**A Survey**

**Please write your answers to the following questions. If you need more space, use the back of the page and write the number of the question along with your answer. Please DO NOT put your name or other identifying information on this survey.**

1.  Please describe the typical ICU patient **before** OIF/OEF. Include age range, typical diagnoses, type of beneficiary (active duty, retired, dependent).

2.  Please describe the typical ICU patient **after the beginning of** OIF/OEF. Include age range, typical diagnoses, type of beneficiary (active duty, retired, dependent).

3.  What were your typical work stressors **before** OIF/OEF?

4.  What are your typical work stressors **since the beginning of** OIF/OEF?

5.  What coping mechanisms did you use to deal with work stressors **before** OIF/OEF?

6.  What coping mechanisms are you currently using **since the beginning of** OIF/OEF?

7.  Is there any other information related to stressors and coping that you would like for us to know?

Fig. 1. ICU nurse questionnaire.

and after OIF and OEF began. ICU head nurses and a critical care clinical nurse specialist validated the stressors and coping mechanisms.

## Patient population

### Average ICU patient before the wars

At most MTFs during peacetime, the mission of the ICU is to care for critically ill military members, their dependents, and a large retiree population. The MTFs also support graduate medical education for physicians in their residency programs. In the civilian sector, 88% of all discharges from ICUs are patients older than 65 years [12]. Although ICU admissions to military MTFs may not reflect this high a number of those older than 65 years, retirees account for a high percentage of ICU admissions during peacetime. Typical diagnoses found in medical ICUs include stroke, acute myocardial infarction, heart failure, respiratory failure, and pneumonia, whereas surgical ICUs consist mostly of patients undergoing cardiovascular procedures [12]. These patient populations are reflected in the ICUs of military MTFs. For this study, nurses at both MTFs described their patient population before the beginning of the war as older (age > 50 years), retired beneficiaries with diagnoses including heart diseases, lung disease, stroke, gastrointestinal bleeds, and those requiring general surgery. Nurses at the MTF in Europe also reported seeing motor vehicle accident victims, because it is a level II trauma center.

### Average ICU patient after the wars

After the beginning of OIF and OEF, the ICUs at these two MTFs assumed very different roles, because medical and surgical treatment primarily involved patients evacuated from the war zones. The average age of ICU patients dropped considerably (to 18–24 years). Primary diagnoses now include polytrauma to major body systems, amputations, and open and closed severe head injuries. Older patients with medical diagnoses are still treated only if room allows, because the injured OIF and OEF patients are given priority over the usual retiree population. Retirees are cared for at local civilian hospitals when the MTF ICUs are filled with injured war fighters.

## Stressors

### Nurse stressors before the wars

Several nurses described their stressors as typical for an ICU: a shortage of nurses and having to work overtime; scheduling conflicts; and communication barriers between doctors, nurses, and leadership personnel. One nurse simply described her stressors as "Code Browns/Code Blues," meaning cleaning up patients who were incontinent of stool (code brown) or resuscitating patients (code blue). Others did not answer this question but provided long answers to the question of stressors after the start of both OIF/OEF.

### Nurse stressors after the beginning of the wars

Shortly after the beginning of OIF and OEF, nursing leadership recognized added stressors when the influx of injured patients began. Two psychiatric clinical nurse specialists in the stateside MTF were instructed to become available to anyone who might need to discuss these added stressors. In the 3 months after the war began in 2003, these clinical nurse specialists saw more than 1000 personnel. Half of these consisted of hospital staff experiencing increased situational stress levels related to wounded soldiers, increased work levels, and reduced staff levels because of deployed colleagues.

Although some nurses described staffing and workload as stressors after the war began, many additional stressors surfaced. Common stressors included the age of the soldiers coupled with the severity of their injuries. One nurse reported "...sadness related to losing young soldiers, dealing with permanent brain damage to young men just beginning [adult] life, young wives having their babies while husband is brain damaged...." Several nurses conveyed distress over issues with the victim's family members, claiming that they were "sometimes too demanding," that "seeing family members' faces as they see their severely injured loved ones for the first time...[b]reaks my heart," and that "Family members deposit their anger upon the nurses like it was our fault that their loved one got wounded." Nurses also expressed great concern over not being able to alleviate their patients' pain. One nurse in the MTF in Europe working in the emergency department became aware of and answered the survey, although she was technically not an ICU nurse. Her anecdote is included because she described how the emergency department became a mini ICU when the ICUs beds were full from the numbers of war injured being evacuated and arriving unexpectedly from the war zones. She presented the prewar stressors as being too many patients seeking nonemergent care and stressing the system, and then described how, after the wars started, nurses in the emergency department were expected to not only care for these critically ill patients as if they were in the ICU but also maintain their usual emergency department patient load. Several nurses, especially those at the MTF in Europe, stated in retrospect that they did not realize how much heavier the workload could get with the flood of wounded warriors. Stressors after the wars began were generally much greater and more diverse than those experienced before the wars. This increased stress level resulted in symptoms among nurses described as *secondary traumatization*, or *compassion fatigue*. The concept of *compassion fatigue* has gained attention within the military health care system as nurses begin to feel overwhelmed by the numbers and types of patients arriving for care.

## The evolution of the concept of vicarious traumatization or compassion fatigue

The term *compassion fatigue* was first used in 1967 to describe the reaction of Americans to the continual calls for donations to the needy [13], and has evolved to include the emotional exhaustion experienced by caregivers. First noted in the nursing literature in 1992, it was described as an exclusive form of burnout that occurs in caregivers as they care for and identify with patients experiencing acute or chronic suffering [14]. In 1995, compassion fatigue was described as a constellation of symptoms resulting from working with trauma victims and vicariously living through the victims' experiences [15]. In 2003, a model was proposed for factors contributing to the development of compassion fatigue, which may be synonymous with *secondary victimization, secondary traumatic stress, vicarious traumatization*, and *secondary posttraumatic stress disorder* [16]. In this model, several factors, including exposure to suffering, empathetic ability, and concern, can predispose one to compassion fatigue, with caregivers experiencing emotional, physical, and spiritual symptoms. These symptoms are strikingly similar to those experienced by individuals diagnosed with posttraumatic stress disorder (PTSD). Symptoms can include

anger, depression, difficulty sleeping, fear, and indifference toward patients as caregivers distance themselves [14,15,17,18].

Before the events of September 11, 2001, most literature discussing compassion fatigue focused on family caregivers of chronically ill patients, such as those who have Alzheimer's disease [19,20]. However, since the 1990s and after the Oklahoma City bombing in 1995, a virtual explosion of literature discusses the effects of traumatic events on counselors and social workers, including the construct of *vicarious traumatization* [21]. As part of this phenomenon, therapists begin to experience feelings and symptoms similar to their clients based on empathetic identification with their situation. After September 11, 2001, a proliferation of writings described the effects on various groups exposed to either the recovery operations or individuals or family members directly involved in the event. From 2002 to 2004, the Mount Sinai School of Medicine evaluated 11,768 workers and volunteers. In a subset of 1138 of these participants, 51% met the threshold criteria of requiring a clinical mental health evaluation and 20% reported symptoms suggestive of PTSD [22].

### Vicarious traumatization applied to nursing

Although little nursing-specific research was found examining compassion fatigue or vicarious traumatization, numerous articles described nurses' stress as related to the care of their patients, especially those who experienced traumatic events. When the variables of emotional contagion, empathic concern, and communicative responsiveness were examined, all were found to significantly explain the variables of depersonalization, reduced personal accomplishment, emotional exhaustion, and reduced occupational commitment [23]. These factors may lead to nurse burnout from a combination of variables impacting this decision, including personal, interpersonal, health care system, and professional [24]. Indirect trauma to nurses and risk factors contributing to the disruption of their sense of well-being has been described [25]. These variables include the type of trauma experienced by patients, the length of the nurse's exposure to patients who have PTSD, the self-efficacy of the nurse, and available support systems. Finally, care must be taken to accurately examine the behavior that makes nurses vulnerable to compassion fatigue: caring [18].

## Deployed versus nondeployed soldiers/nurses

Although some studies describe the stressors of nurses who have deployed to war zones, few describe the stressors and feelings of nurses caring for wounded soldiers who have returned from the war zone for definitive care.

### Deployed nurses

The conditions of nursing care during deployment, such as difficult environmental situations, danger, and atypical situations, place military nurses at risk for moral distress. Working and living under austere and often life-threatening conditions, along with providing nursing care to a constant influx of young traumatically injured soldiers, the environment, and limited available resources, could understandably result in moral distress for deployed nurses. Other risk factors contributing to moral distress may include the sudden and often unexpected order to participate in an imminent military deployment, along with the resulting separation from family and removal from usual support systems. Even under these circumstances, military nurses are still expected to provide expert care [26].

One study identified continual adjustment as a survival mechanism for nurses describing war as a series of ongoing adjustments, which persisted postdeployment [27]. "Living and working during war mandated the types of adjustments in daily living that few nurses anticipated" [27]. They identified innovation and improvisation, social interactions, loyalty, rest and relaxation tours, and keeping journals as coping mechanisms for their difficult situations. Creative talent, including memorializing the experience and friends, was identified as helpful for reentry into postwar life. However, postwar adjustment is not a simple or quick process. "For many, adjustment to civilian life took decades" [27]. One Vietnam nurse veteran stated, "I don't like to be around fatigues [the uniform worn in battle by war fighters at the time of the Vietnam war]. Up until 1984, I could only smell blood around them" [28]. "There … will always be events and places that trigger thoughts of the war. It is unlikely that an individual ever puts war experiences to rest. Waves of involuntary thoughts and feelings always resurface" [28].

### Nondeployed nurses

Very little is recognized or understood about nondeployed soldiers or nurses during major deployment, the government worker whose job is impacted by the situation, or the reservist who is activated to provide support for the continued or changed mission of the facilities. For those unfamiliar with military nursing, most active duty nurses deploy to a war zone sometime during their career, with reserve nurses either "back-filling" the active duty nurse's job or also required to deploy. In the meantime, patient care at the original MTF must continue; hence, civilian government nurses, who do not deploy, are essential to a seamless transition of care. Supporting literature for these unique groups of caregivers who are left behind is limited. A comprehensive literature review found very little addressing the experience of the nondeployed soldier during war. No articles were found that addressed stressors and responses of government workers whose duties are affected by war or for reservists called to active duty for homeland support. Only one study compared symptoms of stress disorders between soldiers who deployed and those who did not [29]. Male military personnel (1187 Canadian peacekeepers versus 669 nondeployed participants) were examined and similar influences of stressors on health in both groups were found, underscoring the need to further study nondeployed personnel. Although the sociodemographic variables of both groups were similar, whether the nondeployed comparison group contained medical personnel or if exposure to traumatized victims occurred could not be determined.

With continued deployments since 2003, large numbers of military nursing personnel are being asked to deploy on short notice. The sudden departure of military nursing personnel is disruptive to the organizational dynamics at the home-station MTF, creating extreme change, stressful and demanding conditions, and requiring high levels of adaptation for the *stay-behind personnel* (eg, nondeployed military nurses, civilian nurses, and activated reservists who support the homeland mission). These groups of nursing personnel must sustain day-to-day operations at their MTFs while often caring for wounded soldiers who are evacuated from the theater of operations.

## Coping mechanisms

### Coping before the wars

The ICU nurses who responded to the questionnaire mentioned several coping mechanisms used before the war. Because the two hospitals were military and many of the nursing staff were soldiers, exercise (which is part of daily life for most military personnel) played a large role in alleviating stress. Other coping mechanisms mentioned included ventilating and debriefing with other coworkers, hobbies, trying to understand their situation, and activities within their social networks. Several nurses stated they did not need coping mechanisms to deal with stress.

*Coping after the beginning of the wars*

Many unique demands and challenges ae associated with military nursing given the contemporary operating environment. Military nurses must endure and manage diverse and significant stressors in the deployed environment and at stateside-based hospitals. Military nurses in various settings and civilian nurses who work in military hospitals are exposed to demanding conditions involving human injury and tragedy. Military and civilian nurses who are indirectly involved with caring for wounded warriors (eg, those participating in case management, administration, education, and research) should also be considered.

The surveyed ICU nurses seemed to use very different coping mechanisms after the beginning of the war. One nurse stated, "Not much ventilation or debrief; we keep information to self; not allowed to comment much about OIF/OEF patients or type of injuries." This same nurse commented that the workload is much greater and there is little time for anything other than patient care (eg, performing collateral duties during periods of low census or acuity). The use of psychiatrists and medication to combat depression increased. Drinking and eating were also used as coping mechanisms among several nurses after the war. Sleeping was mentioned several times as a coping mechanism, although some nurses started dreaming about their patients and needed sleep aids. One nurse who also had combat experience commented about being better able to deal with the stressors because the non–field hospital is a safer environment. Only one nurse mentioned using spirituality as a coping mechanism after the war began.

## Case example of additional support from the medical treatment facility in Europe

In 2005, the Commander of the MTF in Europe contacted a hospital chaplain to ask

what services were available for the ICU staff who had been greatly impacted by the death of a patient. From that event and the actions taken to address the emotional needs of the ICU nurses, it became clear that nurses throughout the facility were experiencing various reactions from direct and indirect exposure to the care of war fighters severely afflicted with or affected by war-related injuries and trauma.

Nurses who had direct exposure were those who provided hands-on patient care and nursing services to wounded warriors. Those who had indirect exposure included mental health staff and indirect caregivers who listened to stories about war-related trauma, human suffering, and grief and loss. Reactions among the nursing staff ranged from minor adjustment problems to physical, emotional, and spiritual distress associated with the difficult work environment, vicarious trauma, or posttrauma.

Commonly reported reactions among nurses who had direct and secondary exposure included not wanting to go to work, difficulty sleeping, feeling tired even with sufficient sleep, increased irritability, anxiety, grief, feeling overwhelmed, lack of motivation, cognitive problems, nausea, and physical fatigue. Risk factors for developing more severe stress responses were direct exposure to severely wounded soldiers on a regular basis, operating under extremely demanding conditions, and dissatisfaction with most aspects of one's career.

The accumulation of work-related (mission-related) or personal stressors contributed to lower adaptability and higher-level symptoms among nursing staff. Those who had previous unresolved grief in addition to the current stressors of caring for the wounded were at greater risk for developing stress reactions.

## Maximizing coping skills

In 2004, just after the beginning of the wars, the Deputy Commander for Nursing Services at the MTF in the United States requested a needs-assessment survey to determine what interventions the nursing staff might use to help them deal with their stressors (Fig. 2). Among those who responded to the survey, 82% (n = 378) expressed a need for personal emotional support. Of those, 49.7% stated they would like in-services for compassion fatigue and PTSD. Another 43.1% requested small informal group sessions where

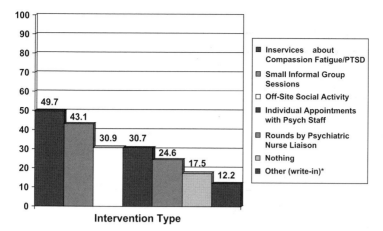

Fig. 2. Caregiver coping needs assessment. *Write-in comments included rest and relaxation (R&R), psychiatric help outside the military system, and bible study.

they could discuss their stressors and learn coping mechanisms.

*Resiliency*

The chaplain at the MTF in Europe noted effective coping skills among nurses who had multiple resources and support systems. Positive interpersonal relationships with coworkers, family members, and friends were protective factors. Finding meaning, purpose, and value in one's work and viewing contributions as important were factors that minimized stress responses. The ability to find positive meaning and experience only temporary disruption in functional capacity and less impact on the body and mind is termed *resilience* [30]. Building resilience increases inner strength and confidence. Resiliency, as experienced by these nurses, permits the will to persevere during complex times and hardships.

The challenge is how to nurture resilience in the nursing community. Two courses of action exist for developing resiliency; a very significant aspect of these is that they are interdependent. The features of one strategy support and enhance the potential for success in the other. The first is the self-care plan and the second is the organizational care plan. A self-care plan is a helpful and productive approach for nurses to deal with the daily stressors of caring for wounded warriors. The self-care plan is developed using the basic foundation of healthy diet, regular exercise, and adequate sleep. From there, individuals can build on their strengths, using all available resources and support systems. Maintaining healthy

relationships and spending time with people who provide positive energy is an important aspect of the self-care plan. Quality time in the family and social settings helps individuals manage and regulate the stressors at work. A healthy balance can also be achieved through various types of leisure and recreational activities.

A very simple but powerful technique for self-care is journal writing. The effectiveness of journal writing is supported by the experience of nurses in the Vietnam war [31]. Journaling helps writers manage feelings and provides a medium for self-reflection. Journaling promotes self-awareness and cultivates insight and wisdom [32].

Recognition and acceptance of all feelings, including uncomfortable and unpleasant ones, is extremely important. Anger, anxiety, sadness, and grief are natural and expected during the lived experience of caring for young patients who have devastating injuries. These feelings can be addressed in a constructive and goal-oriented fashion through journaling or discussion with a trusted individual (eg, friend, family member, colleague, mental health provider, clergy).

Equally as important as the self-care plan is an organizational care plan that integrates the concepts of resiliency. Internal support from within an organization is significant by recognizing its members as valuable and important. Structured support programs in the workplace help individuals and workgroups adapt during adversity.

Staff resiliency programs have an enormous potential to positively affect health and fitness, increase job satisfaction, improve retention, and enhance the overall mission accomplishment through organizational effectiveness and productivity. Although the concept of staff resiliency is somewhat new in military hospital environments, programs for assisting staff and promoting resiliency can only exist when full support is provided by hospital leadership, appropriate resources, and adequate funding [33–38].

In 2005, a support team composed of chaplains, psychiatric nurses, and behavioral health staff was formed at one Army MTF. The team continues to grow and expand its services to support the caregivers and staff impacted by OIF and OEF. The service offers individual consultation for staff members, discussion groups, workshops, presentations, team-building activities, conflict resolution sessions, and consultation with hospital leadership for promoting a positive and supportive work environment.

Programs like these are beginning to emerge throughout the Army, with the recognition that support for caregivers is essential to maximize patient outcomes and mitigate the effects of compassion fatigue. Although research-based data on use and efficacy are not available because of the early stages of these programs, the following lessons have been learned about development, team structure, and delivery of services: (1) interprofessional team membership provides the opportunity for collegial and professional sharing, (2) interprofessional team membership provides a broad knowledge base, (3) a structured and methodical approach with regular team meetings, discussions, and brainstorming is necessary for program success, (4) marketing, visibility, and easy access are factors that increase program use, (5) offering a variety of services is more effective than providing a single type of service, (6) it is important to accommodate shift workers.

## Summary

It is evident that the "stay behind" nurses at both MTFs have experienced significant stress from (1) the deployment of colleagues and, in some cases, family members; (2) changing missions related to the care of wounded soldiers returning to the medical center; and (3) the extra work created by deployments, with few backfill replacements, and the influx of younger patients who have increased levels of acuity and need. It is also evident that resiliency programs can have a positive effect in nurses' coping mechanisms, as demonstrated by their implementation within one

of the Army's MTFs. Because of increased stressors such as those experienced by the critical care nurses surveyed, and the need for both reactive and preventative interventions, further study of both compassion fatigue and resiliency as phenomena is needed in more military MTFs.

## References

[1] Schwam K. The phenomenon of compassion fatigue in perioperative nursing. AORN J 1998; 68(4):642–8.

[2] Levy MM. Caring for the caregiver. Crit Care Clin 2004;20:541–7.

[3] Stehle JL. Critical care nursing stress: the findings revisited. Nurs Res 1981;30:182–7.

[4] Keane A, Ducette J, Adler DC. Stress in ICU and non-ICU nurses. Nurs Res 1985;34:231–6.

[5] Tummers GER, van Merode GG, Landeweerd JA. The diversity of work: differences, similarities and relationships concerning characteristics of the organization, the work and psychological work reactions in intensive care and non-intensive care nursing. Int J Nurs Stud 2002;39:841–55.

[6] Meltzer LS, Huckabay LM. Critical care nurses' perceptions of futile care and its effect on burnout. Am J Crit Care 2004;13:202–8.

[7] Jezuit DL. Suffering of critical care nurses with end-of-life decisions. Medsurg Nurs 2000;9:145–52.

[8] Badger JM. A descriptive study of coping strategies used by medical intensive care unit nurses during transitions from cure- to comfort-oriented care. Heart Lung 2004;34:63–8.

[9] Brosche TA. A grief team within a healthcare system. Dimens Crit Care Nurs 2007;26(1):21–8.

[10] Smith AM, Ortiguera SA, Laskowski ER, et al. A preliminary analysis of psychophysiological variables and nursing performance in situations of increasing criticality. Mayo Clin Proc 2001;76: 275–84.

[11] Elpern EH, Covert B, Kleinpell R. Moral distress of staff nurses in a medical intensive care unit. Am J Crit Care 2005;14:523–30.

[12] Cooper LM, Linde-Zwirble WT. Medical intensive care unit use: analysis of incidence, cost, and payment. Crit Care Med 2004;32:2247–52.

[13] Farmer AW. The national director of CWS appeals. The Vidette Messenger 1967. Available at: http://www.phrases.org.uk/meanings/compassion-fatigue.html. Accessed June 6, 2007.

[14] Joinson C. Coping with compassion fatigue. Nursing 1992;22(4):116–21.

[15] Adams RE, Boscarino JA, Figley CR. Compassion fatigue and psychological distress among social workers: a validation study. Am J Orthopsychiatry 2006;76:103–8.

[16] Figley CR. Compassion fatigue: an introduction. Green Cross Foundation; 2003. Available at:

www.greencross.org/_Research/Compassionfatigue. asp. Accessed February 19, 2005.

[17] Figley CR. Chart 2: examples of compassion fatigue burnout symptoms. 2005. Available at: http:// mailer.fsu.edu/%7ecfigley/CFChart.html. Retrieved February 19, 2005.

[18] Sabo BM. Compassion fatigue and nursing work: can we accurately capture the consequences of caring work? Int J Nurs Pract 2006;12:136–42.

[19] Drebing CE. Trends in the content and methodology of Alzheimer caregiving research. Alzheimer Dis Assoc Disord 1999;13:S93–100.

[20] McCarty EF, Drebing CE. Burden and professional caregivers: tracking the impact. J Nurses Staff Dev 2002;18(5):250–7.

[21] Sexton L. Vicarious traumatisation of counselors and effects on their workplaces. Br J Guid Counc 1999;27(3):393–402.

[22] Center for Disease Control. Mental health status of World Trade Center rescue and recovery workers and volunteers, New York City, July 2002–August 2004. MMWR CDC Surveill Summ 2004;53(35): 812–5.

[23] Omdahl BL, O'Donnell C. Emotional contagion, empathic concern and communicative responsiveness as variables affecting nurses' stress and occupational commitment. J Adv Nurs 1999;29(6):1351–9.

[24] Sherman DW. Palliative nursing: nurses' stress & burnout: how to care for yourself when caring for patients and their families experiencing life-threatening illness. Am J Nurs 2004;104(5):48–57.

[25] Clark ML, Gioro S. Nurses, indirect trauma, and prevention. Image J Nurs Scholarsh 1998;30(1):85–7.

[26] Fry S, Harvey R, Hurley A, et al. Development of a model of moral distress in military nursing. Nurs Ethics 2002;9(4):373–87.

[27] Stanton MP, Dittmar SS, Jezewski MA, et al. Shared experiences and meanings of military nurse veterans. Image J Nurs Sch 1996;28(4):343–7.

[28] Norman E. Women at war: the story of fifty military nurses who served in Vietnam. Philadelphia: University of Pennsylvania Press; 1990. p. 150–1.

[29] Asmundson GJ, Stein MB, McCreary DR. Posttraumatic stress disorder symptoms influence health status of deployed peacekeepers and nondeployed military personnel [Comparative Study. Journal Article]. J Nerv Ment Dis 2002;190(12):807–15.

[30] Bonanno GA. Loss, trauma and human resilience: have we underestimated the human capacity to thrive after extremely aversive events? Am Psychol 2004;59(1):20–8.

[31] Scannell-Desch EA. The lived experience of women military nurses in Vietnam during the Vietnam War. Image J Nurs Sch 1996;28(2):119–24.

[32] Mulligan L. Overcoming compassion fatigue [Journal Article, Pictorial]. Kans Nurse 2004;79(7):1–2.

[33] Hays MA, All AC, Mannahan C, et al. Reported stressors and ways of coping utilized by intensive care unit nurses. Dimens Crit Care Nurs 2006; 25(4):185–93.

[34] Gutierrez KM. Critical care nurses' perceptions and responses to moral distress. Dimens Crit Care Nurs 2005;24(5):229–41.

[35] Jezuit DL. The manager's role during nurse suffering: creating an environment of support and compassion. JONAS Healthc Law Ethics Regul 2002; 4(5):26–9.

[36] Jones MC, Johnston DW. A critical review of the relationship between perception of the work environment, coping and mental health in trained nurses, and patient outcomes. Clinical Effectiveness in Nursing 2000;4:75–85.

[37] Rushton CH. Defining and addressing moral distress: tools for critical care nursing leaders. AACN Adv Crit Care 2006;17(2):161–8.

[38] Collins S, Long A. Too tired to care? The psychological effects of working with trauma. J Psychiatr Ment Health Nurs 2003;10:17–27.

ELSEVIER
SAUNDERS

Crit Care Nurs Clin N Am 20 (2008) 51–57

CRITICAL CARE
NURSING CLINICS
OF NORTH AMERICA

# Pain Management in the Traumatic Amputee

## Ann Kobiela Ketz, MN, RN, AOCNS, CPT, AN, USA[a,b,*]

[a]Department of Emergency Medicine, Landstuhl Regional Medical Center,
CMR 402 Box 512, APO AE 09180, Landstuhl, Germany
[b]212th Combat Support Hospital, CMR 403, APO AE 09059 Miesau, Germany

## Traumatic amputations

Combat operations in Operation Enduring Freedom (OEF) and Operation Iraqi Freedom (OIF) have left at least 562 members of the United States Armed Service without limbs. This loss of limbs, not including fingers or toes, accounts for a total major amputation rate of 2.27% of all casualties as of March 1, 2007 [1]. Advances in military medicine, such as far-forward surgical intervention, improved surgical techniques, and quick evacuation to tertiary care facilities, together with improved protective gear, have resulted in lower casualty and amputation rates than in previous conflicts [2].

Most orthopedic combat injuries are associated with fragmentation of ordnance and landmines [3–5]. Many landmines or suicide bombs are improvised explosive devices (IEDs) that may be composed of nails, bolts, and shards of glass. Wounds inflicted by IEDs often are contaminated by dirt and pieces of clothing or bone [6].

Traumatic amputations are not only a concern for the military. The United Nations reports more than 250,000 amputees worldwide in its registry [7]. Currently, there are more than 80 million landmines buried worldwide in at least 84 countries [7–9], most from previous or ongoing military conflicts, putting civilians at risk for traumatic amputations. Motor vehicle crashes and machinery accidents also can cause traumatic injuries requiring amputation. Regardless of the cause of the injury, traumatic amputations result in complex pain management issues. Persons whose traumatic amputations are considered "dirty," as from IEDs, may experience painful serial wound irrigations, dressing changes, and placement of instruments to stabilize fractures [2,10]. Postamputation pain can influence patients' mobility, sleep, and overall quality of life [11]. The purpose of this article is (1) to describe the current evidence as it seeks to explain the pathophysiology of the types of pain resulting from limb amputations and (2) to explain the best practices in treatment options.

### Phantom limb pain

After the amputation of a limb, patients commonly experience persistent sensations in the removed limb [12]. They may experience phantom sensation, characterized by feeling the missing limb's position in space, touch, pressure, temperature, itching, tingling, wetness, sweatiness, and other nonpainful sensations [13]. In addition to phantom sensations, 50% to 80% of amputation patients report pain in the amputated limb [12,14]. This phantom limb pain (PLP) has been described by patients as "stabbing" (24.3%) or "pins and needles" (20.5%) [12], although the pain experience can be unique to each amputee. The onset of PLP may be immediate following an amputation, and in some cases PLP can last throughout the amputee's life. Although many individuals who have PLP report it as being mild and intermittent, it may be severe enough to interfere with a patient's work, sleep, and social life [11–13].

The views expressed in this manuscript are those of the authors and do not reflect the official policy of the Department of Army, the Department of Defense, or US Government.

* Department of Emergency Medicine, Landstuhl Regional Medical Center, CMR 402 Box 512, APO AE 09180, Landstuhl, Germany.

E-mail addresses: ann.kobiela.ketz@us.army.mil; annketz@googlemail.com

## Residual limb pain

Amputees also can experience pain in the remaining stump or residual limb. Residual limb pain (RLP) is caused most often by neuroma formation. Neuromas are bulb-shaped thickenings formed by abnormal regrowth of nerve fibers after traumatic or surgical injury [15]. This abnormal growth of the nerve fibers can produce irregular activity that causes pain by stimulating central neurons. Phantom sensation, PLP, and RLP can be experienced separately or may be related [16], contributing to the challenge of differentiating and treating appropriately the pain experienced by amputees regardless of the cause or location.

For patients wounded in combat situations, specifically in OEF/OIF, traumatic amputations rarely occur as an isolated injury. Common associated painful injuries of amputees from OEF/OIF include multiple limb amputations (16%), long bone fractures (39%), active infections (45%), other soft tissue injuries (41%), and peripheral nerve injuries (12%) [17]. Additionally, these traumatic amputees may suffer pain related to heterotopic ossification, or the growth of mature lamellar bone in nonbone tissue, usually of the residual limb [18,19]. Many amputees reporting PLP and RLP also experience pain at sites including, but not limited to, the back, unaffected leg/foot, buttocks/hips, neck/shoulders, and arms/hands. Over one third (36%) of a sample of 57 amputees experienced PLP, RLP, and back pain [20]. These injuries increase the burden of pain and contribute to the overall complexity in the care of these patients.

Several causative factors, both peripheral and central, may contribute to PLP, but the exact etiology is yet unknown [21]. Reorganization of the cortex of the brain following amputations may contribute to PLP [21,22]. Another theory considers both peripheral and central factors. Melzack [13,23] has described the "neuromatrix" as a neuronal network of combined somatosensory, limbic (emotional), and cognitive circuitry that together represents the integrated body experience, or "self." This subjective body experience may remain intact even after a body part has been removed surgically, and therefore the patient may still experience pain and other sensations in the absent body part.

The complex etiology of PLP lends to a variety of problems, including the potential for underreporting of pain in suffering patients. In a survey of 2694 military veterans, only 54% reporting PLP sought treatment from their health care provider, and only 19% of those patients were offered any treatment [14]. A similar study conducted in England reported that only 72 of 526 PLP sufferers requested any treatment from their health care provider [12]. In both surveys, individual patients reported being told that there was nothing their health care provider could do for their pain or that the pain should resolve on its own. Several patients stated that their health care providers avoided answering the questions or told them that the pain was only "in their head" [12,14]. These reports are not surprising, considering the lack of evidence from controlled, long-term studies with large sample sizes and adequate follow-up that show effective treatments for PLP.

## Treatments

Although few well-controlled trials have addressed the treatment of postamputation pain, there are published case reports describing isolated episodes of pain control or complete relief achieved by a wide variety of modalities, such as methadone [24], hypnosis [25], electromyography and biofeedback [26], and the use of a specialized prosthesis [27]. Treatments, including local anesthesia, sympathectomy, dorsal-root entry-zone lesions, cordotomy, neurostimulation methods, and pharmacologic interventions such as anticonvulsants, barbiturates, antidepressants, neuroleptics, and muscle relaxants, have been beneficial only 30% of the time, similar to the placebo effect reported in different studies [21]. Investigators continue to search for ways to treat postamputation pain consistently.

## Prevention

Patients may experience "pain memory," a phenomenon in which painful phantom sensations mimic the pain felt before amputation [28]. Pain memory, along with theories of cortical reorganization resulting in PLP, has led researchers to hypothesize that preamputation pain may influence PLP [29,30], and others have suggested the importance of pain management before and immediately after amputation surgeries [31]. Lower limb amputees (70% traumatic) who received perioperative epidural analgesia were interviewed before amputation, immediately postoperatively, and at 6, 12, and 24 months following amputation. They found that the intensity of preamputation pain significantly predicted the intensity of acute (4–5 days postoperative) PLP ($P < .01$) and long-term (24-month postoperative) PLP ($P < .05$). The intensity of acute PLP significantly predicted the intensity of PLP 6 and 12 months postoperatively ($P < .01$ and $.001$, respectively), but not of 24-month PLP. They found similar results with RLP, indicating that both preamputation and acute pain may predict chronic pain [31]. These results emphasize the importance of preventing preoperative and acute postoperative pain.

Attempts to prevent postamputation RLP and PLP have produced conflicting results [32–35]. Patients who received pre-, peri- and postoperative epidural bupivacaine, morphine, and clonidine had significantly less PLP at 1 year than those who received opioids only postoperatively ($P < .002$). In a randomized, double-blind trial, epidural bupivacaine and morphine administered 18 hours pre- and perioperatively did not prevent acute or chronic RLP or PLP [32]. Another study compared postamputation pain in patients randomly assigned to receive epidural bupivacaine and diamorphine from 24 hours preoperatively to 3 days postoperatively or perineural bupivacaine peri- and postoperatively. The results indicated no significant benefit for preoperative epidural bupivacaine and diamorphine in preventing PLP, although it did relieve acute RLP significantly [33]. Similarly, a cross-sectional survey comparing pain interviews from 1 week to 14 months following amputation found no significant differences in chronic pain among patients who received epidural, spinal, or general anesthesia, although patients who received epidural or spinal anesthesia reported significantly less acute pain than those who received general anesthesia. There was no difference between the three groups in the postoperative use of pain medication [34]. Given the potential link between preamputation and acute pain and chronic RLP and PLP, further studies are warranted to determine ways to prevent early pain in high-risk patients.

## Medications

Gabapentin, originally an antiepileptic drug, has been recommended as adjuvant treatment for neuropathic pain syndromes [36,37]. Two prominent double-blind, placebo-controlled, crossover trials examining the efficacy of gabapentin for PLP report conflicting results. One study revealed a decrease in spontaneous PLP after 6 weeks of treatment with gabapentin (300–2400 mg) but no change in secondary outcome indices of sleep interference, mood, and activities of daily living [36]. Other investigators measured the average and worst PLP and RLP intensity on a 0-to-10 numeric rating scale and secondarily measured the meaningfulness of changes in pain from pre- to posttreatment [37]. There were no significant differences in PLP or RLP intensity in the gabapentin phase (300–3600 mg) versus the placebo phase, although significantly more patients reported meaningful decreases in pain during the gabapentin phase than in the placebo phase ($P < .05$). Along with the conflicting outcomes, the fact that both studies were underpowered indicates that further studies are warranted to determine the efficacy of gabapentin for PLP and RLP. Another study compared gabapentin with placebo for 30 days postoperatively in a sample of elderly patients who had amputations because pf peripheral vascular disease. This study also found no significant differences in short- or long-term (6 months) pain measurement [38]. Future studies should include larger samples of both traumatic and nontraumatic amputees and focus on consistent outcome measures to allow comparison.

Amputees have reported high helpfulness ratings [39] and patient satisfaction [12] from the use of opioids to manage postamputation pain, even though few randomized, controlled trials have studied the efficacy of opioid use for PLP. Methadone was used to reduce PLP intensity successfully in four patients when other drugs, including other opioids, were unsuccessful [24]. The effect of oral morphine on PLP was studied in a sample of 12 unilateral amputees reporting PLP intensity of 3 or higher out of 10 on a visual analog scale (VAS) in a randomized, double-blind, placebo-controlled cross-over design study [40]. Investigators measured pain by VAS recordings in a pain diary and measured sensory and affective dimensions of pain with the pain-experience scale (PES). Pain diaries showed significantly less pain intensity in the treatment phase than in either the baseline ($P < .01$) or the placebo phases ($P = .036$). PES measures indicated significantly less pain in the treatment phase than in the baseline (affective: $P < .01$; sensory: $P < .001$) or placebo (affective: $P < .001$; sensory: $P < .01$) phases. Participants who demonstrated a clinically relevant response (eg, pain reduction of more than 50%) in the 4-week treatment phase (n = 9) were maintained on long-term oral morphine for pain management

(70–300 mg/d by 12-month follow-up). Follow-up at 6 and 12 months demonstrated a significant main effect for both pain diary ratings ($P < .01$) and the PES-sensory pain scale ($P < .05$) [40].

The use of opioids for chronic, and especially neuropathic, pain remains controversial. Many traumatic amputees are young, otherwise healthy individuals who need to maintain high levels of functioning in their personal and professional lives. Both patients and health care providers may have concerns about opioids' negative side-effect profile, including gastrointestinal and cognitive effects, as well as fears of addiction or dependence [41].

## Surgical treatments

Interventional therapies, such as perineural nerve blocks, have been used successfully to alleviate acute postoperative PLP but have had conflicting results in preventing or relieving chronic PLP [42–44]. A simple surgical intervention has been developed that has shown promise in reducing phantom sensation and pain in lower limb amputees, however [45]. The technique involves dissecting the sciatic nerve, reattaching the halves in a sling fashion, and covering the nerve with a fibrin patch. Ropivacaine then is administered postoperatively for 5 days at the surgical site. In this small study (n = 15), results showed that average, maximum, and minimum pain intensity scores were significantly reduced at 1 week, 3 months, 6 months, and 1 year after surgery ($P < .001$) [45]. The majority of participants had amputations from a nontraumatic cause (n = 14), so this study should be replicated in a larger sample that includes traumatic amputees.

Surgical treatments also have been used to manage RLP caused by neuroma formation. Current strategies include implanting the nerve ending into muscle or bone tissue, using nonvascular autologous or synthetic materials to construct a cap for the nerve ending, or capping the nerve with vascular soft tissue [15,46].

## Complementary and alternative treatments

Certain nonstandard therapies have shown potential effectiveness in relieving, and even eliminating, PLP in several published case reports and small studies. Therefore these therapies may be used in addition to or instead of standard medical pain treatments.

Anecdotal observations from one military health care facility report amputees had pain relief lasting hours to days after receiving ear and/or scalp acupuncture, allowing them to participate in rehabilitation and experience better sleep [10]. The benefits of ear and scalp acupuncture include its ease of application in outpatient and bedside settings, lack of interference with traditional rehabilitation, and the ease of implementation by providers without prior experience [10]. A case study of three patients suffering from PLP who received acupuncture to their intact limb demonstrated complete relief of PLP after treatment in two of the three patients [47]. Ten-minute auricular transcutaneous electrical nerve stimulation sessions resulted in a statistically significant ($P < .01$) but modest short-term decrease in PLP when measured by the McGill Pain Questionnaire [48].

One case report describes using a combination of electromyography and thermal biofeedback to treat PLP in an upper extremity. The participant had been experiencing PLP since 1 month after his amputation, which had occurred 3 years before treatment. He reported pretreatment PLP intensity of 8 on a 0 (no pain)-to-10 (intolerable pain) VAS and described burning and shooting pain, as well as coldness in his hand. After two sessions to collect baseline data, he participated in six sessions each of exercises to manipulate tension in the stump and to raise stump temperature. Mean skin temperature and electromyography were measured in the stump and the intact arm and were compared. The participant continued to apply the temperature biofeedback strategies following treatment. He reported a PLP score of 3 on the VAS at the end of treatment and no pain at both the 3-and 12-month follow-up interviews [26].

Hypnosis and imagery techniques also have been used to treat cases of PLP, based on the theory that suggestion and imagery may have an effect in the areas of the brain involved in pain perception [49,50]. One case describes a man whose upper extremity was amputated following an avulsion of his brachial plexus. His PLP was relieved while he viewed his "arms" in a Ramachandran mirror apparatus, in which the intact arm is placed inside a mirrored box, and the image is reflected to appear as bilateral intact arms [51]; however, his pain level increased within an hour after using the apparatus. The authors then led him through an eyes-closed hypnotic induction and deepening, during which they asked him to "see" his arms in the mirror apparatus. The man again reported relief from his pain, but, unfortunately, no short- or long-term follow-up was recorded [25]. Other case reports report up to 55% reduction in PLP frequency in traumatic amputees after hypnosis sessions [52].

Energy-healing therapies are based on the concept that human beings have a subtle energy field that can be manipulated to effect changes in the body and influence health. One of the most commonly studied energy-healing therapies in scientific literature is therapeutic touch (TT). The concept of TT has been used in Eastern healing since ancient times and was introduced to American nursing 30 years ago by Dolores Krieger and Dora Kunz [53–55]. The premise of TT is the belief that a universal energy, or "life force," sustains all living things [56] and that each person's "human field image" is pandimensional and extends beyond the physical body [57]. In the practice of TT, the practitioner serves as a channel for the universal healing energy to affect the entire field of the patient [56]. Several published case studies report relief from PLP after TT treatments, including a World War II veteran who had been suffering from PLP for 40 years [57]. Studying the impact of TT on pain relief in randomized, controlled trials is, understandably, challenging, but several successful attempts have been made. A single blind, randomized, controlled experimental pilot study was conducted to determine the effect of TT on amputees who had PLP and/or RLP. Nine patients were assigned to a control, placebo, or treatment group for 12 sessions. Patients in the control group received no TT, the placebo group received mimic TT, and the treatment group received actual TT. The investigators used a vertical VAS to measure both pain and well being and observed vital signs immediately before, immediately after, and 1 hour after the session. Although no significant changes in vital signs occurred, pain scale measurements showed a 75% reduction in pain scores from immediately before to immediately after treatment; this change was significant when compared with the other groups ($P = .0001$). The results from 1 hour after treatment did not reach significance, however [56]. This study was conducted in an inpatient rehabilitation setting, so the results cannot be generalized to the outpatient setting.

Anecdotally, amputees have been known to wrap their residual limbs in aluminum foil in an attempt to reduce PLP. Based on this observation, a double-blind, randomized, cross-over study was designed in which patients who reported mild to severe PLP ($\geq 3$ on a 0–10 pain scale) wore a metal stump liner interwoven with electromagnetically shielding properties [58]. After collecting 2 weeks of baseline data, the 30 participants were fitted for a silicone stocking. Half received the experimental liner, and half received a dummy liner. Two weeks later, the participants received the opposite liner to wear for an additional 2 weeks. The investigators measured PLP six times daily with a 1-to-10 numeric rating scale, along with once-daily assessments of improvement in well-being and sleep. Participants reported significant decreases in the duration of both chronic PLP ($P = .008$) and maximum PLP ($P = .031$) levels when wearing the experimental liner versus the placebo liner. Calculated odd ratios indicated that participants were more likely to have decreased chronic and maximum PLP when wearing the experimental liner (odds ratios, 5.95 and 4.5, respectively). Wearing the experimental liner also improved well-being measures significantly over the placebo liner ($P < .001$). Although measures for sleep quality were not significantly different between the experimental and the placebo liner, the investigators did find that the participants voluntarily wore the experimental liner at night twice as much as the placebo liner [58].

Complementary and alternative medicine treatments must be studied more thoroughly to determine their effectiveness in relieving pain in amputees. They do not have the same risk for side effects and addiction or dependence as opioids, antidepressants, and anticonvulsants [25,47,56]. The lack of side effects and addiction risk with complementary and alternative medicine therapies are attractive for patients who are highly functional and active, such as amputees from combat in OEF/OIF.

### Self-treatment

In addition to standard surgical, medical, and complementary and alternative medicine treatments for chronic pain, many amputees find self-treatment pain relief methods that work for them. These treatments may include residual limb tapping, massage, towel pulls, desensitization, distraction, meditation, and alcohol/drug use. Because PLP often is intermittent, these types of treatments may be all that an amputee needs to manage pain. The effectiveness of self-care methods has not been examined in any detail in the literature, although several studies mention self-care and coping methods used by patients suffering from PLP such as distraction, stump manipulation, exercise, and alcohol and marijuana use [12,14,16]. Results from these studies report high variability in the relief of PLP provided by these methods, and further research must be done to determine their efficacy and clinical significance in improving patient outcomes.

## Summary

PLP and RLP related to traumatic amputations will continue to be a problem for the military health care system and international medical community as well as negatively influencing amputees' quality of life. The disparity between what is known about the causes and treatments for PLP and RLP and current practice must be addressed to improve outcomes for patients who suffer from postamputation pain. Health care providers must place a priority on continuing to assess pain issues throughout the continuum of care. Providers at every level of care should be informed about the multitude of treatment options that exist, and about emerging research, to ensure that patients receive the individualized pain management that they deserve.

## References

[1] Amputee monthly statistics. The United States Armed Forces Amputee Patient Care Program; March 1, 2007.

[2] Smith DG, Granville RR. Moderators' summary: amputee care. J Am Acad Orthop Surg 2006; 14(Suppl 10):S179–82.

[3] Husum H, Gilbert M, Wisborg T, et al. Land mine injuries: a study of 708 victims in North Iraq and Cambodia. Mil Med 2003;168(11):934–40.

[4] Islinger RB, Kuklo TR, McHale KA. A review of orthopedic injuries in three recent U.S. military conflicts. Mil Med 2000;165(6):463–5.

[5] Jovanovic S, Wertheimer B, Zelic Z, et al. Wartime amputations. Mil Med 1999;164(1):44–7.

[6] Gawande A. Casualties of war—military care for the wounded from Iraq and Afghanistan. N Engl J Med 2004;351(24):2471–5.

[7] Landmines factsheet. Available at: http://www.un.org/cyberschoolbus/banmines/facts.asp. Accessed November 29, 2004.

[8] O'Brien E. The land mine crisis: a growing epidemic of mutilation. Lancet 1994;vol 344:1522.

[9] Landmine facts. Available at: http://www.un.org/Depts/dha/mct/facts.htm. Accessed April 27, 2007.

[10] Niemtzow RC, Gambel J, Helms J, et al. Integrating ear and scalp acupuncture techniques into the care of blast-injured United States military service members with limb loss. J Altern Complement Med 2006; 12(7):596–9.

[11] Sherman RA. Utilization of prostheses among US veterans with traumatic amputation: a pilot survey. J Rehabil Res Dev 1999;36(2):100–8.

[12] Wartan SW, Hamann W, Wedley JR, et al. Phantom pain and sensation among British veteran amputees. Br J Anaesth 1997;78(6):652–9.

[13] Melzack R. Phantom limbs and the concept of a neuromatrix. Trends Neurosci 1990;13(3):88–92.

[14] Sherman RA, Sherman CJ, Parker L. Chronic phantom and stump pain among American veterans: results of a survey. Pain 1984;18(1):83–95.

[15] Lewin-Kowalik J, Marcol W, Kotulska K, et al. Prevention and management of painful neuroma. Neurol Med Chir (Tokyo) 2006;46(2):62–7 [discussion 67–68].

[16] Whyte AS, Niven CA. Variation in phantom limb pain: results of a diary study. J Pain Symptom Manage 2001;22(5):947–53.

[17] Potter BK, Scoville CR. Amputation is not isolated: an overview of the US army amputee patient care program and associated amputee injuries. J Am Acad Orthop Surg 2006;14(Suppl 10):S188–90.

[18] Potter BK, Burns TC, Lacap AP, et al. Heterotopic ossification in the residual limbs of traumatic and combat-related amputees. J Am Acad Orthop Surg 2006;14(Suppl 10):S191–7.

[19] Potter BK, Burns TC, Lacap AP, et al. Heterotopic ossification following traumatic and combat-related amputations. Prevalence, risk factors, and preliminary results of excision. J Bone Joint Surg Am 2007;89(3):476–86.

[20] Ehde DM, Czerniecki JM, Smith DG, et al. Chronic phantom sensations, phantom pain, residual limb pain, and other regional pain after lower limb amputation. Arch Phys Med Rehabil 2000;81(8):1039–44.

[21] Flor H. Phantom-limb pain: characteristics, causes, and treatment. Lancet Neurol 2002;1(3):182–9.

[22] Flor H, Nikolajsen L, Staehelin Jensen T. Phantom limb pain: a case of maladaptive CNS plasticity? Nat Rev Neurosci 2006;7(11):873–81.

[23] Melzack R. Pain and the neuromatrix in the brain. J Dent Educ 2001;65(12):1378–82.

[24] Bergmans L, Snijdelaar DG, Katz J, et al. Methadone for phantom limb pain. Clin J Pain 2002; 18(3):203–5.

[25] Oakley DA, Whitman LG, Halligan PW. Hypnotic imagery as a treatment for phantom limb pain: two case reports and a review. Clin Rehabil 2002;16(4): 368–77.

[26] Belleggia G, Birbaumer N. Treatment of phantom limb pain with combined EMG and thermal biofeedback: a case report. Appl Psychophysiol Biofeedback 2001;26(2):141–6.

[27] Weiss T, Miltner WH, Adler T, et al. Decrease in phantom limb pain associated with prosthesis-induced increased use of an amputation stump in humans. Neurosci Lett 1999;272(2):131–4.

[28] Katz J, Melzack R. Pain 'memories' in phantom limbs: review and clinical observations. Pain 1990; 43(3):319–36.

[29] Nikolajsen L, Ilkjaer S, Kroner K, et al. The influence of preamputation pain on postamputation stump and phantom pain. Pain 1997;72(3):393–405.

[30] Jensen TS, Krebs B, Nielsen J, et al. Immediate and long-term phantom limb pain in amputees: incidence, clinical characteristics and relationship to pre-amputation limb pain. Pain 1985;21(3):267–78.

[31] Hanley MA, Jensen MP, Smith DG, et al. Preamputation pain and acute pain predict chronic pain after lower extremity amputation. J Pain 2007;8(2):102–9 Epub 2006 Sep 2001.

[32] Nikolajsen L, Ilkjaer S, Christensen JH, et al. Randomised trial of epidural bupivacaine and morphine in prevention of stump and phantom pain in lower-limb amputation. Lancet 1997;350(9088):1353–7.

[33] Lambert AW, Dashfield AK, Cosgrove C, et al. Randomized prospective study comparing preoperative epidural and intraoperative perineural analgesia for the prevention of postoperative stump and phantom limb pain following major amputation. Reg Anesth Pain Med 2001;26(4):316–21.

[34] Ong BY, Arneja A, Ong EW. Effects of anesthesia on pain after lower-limb amputation. J Clin Anesth 2006;18(8):600–4.

[35] Jahangiri M, Jayatunga AP, Bradley JW, et al. Prevention of phantom pain after major lower limb amputation by epidural infusion of diamorphine, clonidine and bupivacaine. Ann R Coll Surg Engl 1994;76(5):324–6.

[36] Bone M, Critchley P, Buggy DJ. Gabapentin in postamputation phantom limb pain: a randomized, double-blind, placebo-controlled, cross-over study. Reg Anesth Pain Med 2002;27(5):481–6.

[37] Smith DG, Ehde DM, Hanley MA, et al. Efficacy of gabapentin in treating chronic phantom limb and residual limb pain. J Rehabil Res Dev 2005;42(5): 645–54.

[38] Nikolajsen L, Finnerup NB, Kramp S, et al. A randomized study of the effects of gabapentin on postamputation pain. Anesthesiology 2006;105(5): 1008–15.

[39] Hanley MA, Ehde DM, Campbell KM, et al. Self-reported treatments used for lower-limb phantom pain: descriptive findings. Arch Phys Med Rehabil 2006;87(2):270–7.

[40] Huse E, Larbig W, Flor H, et al. The effect of opioids on phantom limb pain and cortical reorganization. Pain 2001;90(1–2):47–55.

[41] Gordon DB, Love G. Pharmacologic management of neuropathic pain. Pain Manag Nurs 2004;5(4, Suppl 1):19–33.

[42] Pinzur MS, Garla PG, Pluth T, et al. Continuous postoperative infusion of a regional anesthetic after an amputation of the lower extremity. A randomized clinical trial. J Bone Joint Surg Am 1996;78(10): 1501–5.

[43] Fisher A, Meller Y. Continuous postoperative regional analgesia by nerve sheath block for amputation surgery—a pilot study. Anesth Analg 1991; 72(3):300–3.

[44] Halbert J, Crotty M, Cameron ID. Evidence for the optimal management of acute and chronic phantom pain: a systematic review. Clin J Pain 2002;18(2): 84–92.

[45] Prantl L, Schreml S, Heine N, et al. Surgical treatment of chronic phantom limb sensation and limb pain after lower limb amputation. Plast Reconstr Surg 2006;118(7):1562–72.

[46] Krishnan KG, Pinzer T, Schackert G. Coverage of painful peripheral nerve neuromas with vascularized soft tissue: method and results. Neurosurgery 2005; 56(Suppl 2):369–78 [discussion 369–78].

[47] Bradbrook D. Acupuncture treatment of phantom limb pain and phantom limb sensation in amputees. Acupunct Med 2004;22(2):93–7.

[48] Katz J, Melzack R. Auricular transcutaneous electrical nerve stimulation (TENS) reduces phantom limb pain. J Pain Symptom Manage 1991;6(2): 73–83.

[49] Willoch F, Rosen G, Tolle TR, et al. Phantom limb pain in the human brain: unraveling neural circuitries of phantom limb sensations using positron emission tomography. Ann Neurol 2000;48(6):842–9.

[50] Rainville P, Duncan GH, Price DD, et al. Pain affect encoded in human anterior cingulate but not somatosensory cortex. Science 1997;277(5328):968–71.

[51] Ramachandran VS, Hirstein W. The perception of phantom limbs. The D.O. Hebb lecture. Brain 1998;121(Pt 9):1603–30.

[52] Rosen G, Willoch F, Bartenstein P, et al. Neurophysiological processes underlying the phantom limb pain experience and the use of hypnosis in its clinical management: an intensive examination of two patients. Int J Clin Exp Hypn 2001;49(1):38–55.

[53] Kunz D, Krieger D. The spiritual dimension of therapeutic touch. Rochester (VT): Bear & Company; 2004.

[54] Krieger D. Therapeutic touch: two decades of research, teaching and clinical practice. Imprint 1990;37(3):83, 86–88.

[55] Krieger D. Alternative medicine: therapeutic touch. Nurs Times 1976;72(15):572–4.

[56] Philcox P, Rawlins L, Rodgers L. Therapeutic touch and its effects on phantom limb and stump pain. Co-operative Connection: Newsletter of the Nurse Healers Professional Associates International, Inc. 2003. p. 24.

[57] Biley FC. Rogerian science, phantoms, and therapeutic touch: exploring potentials. Nurs Sci Q 1996;9(4):165–9.

[58] Kern U, Altkemper B, Kohl M. Management of phantom pain with a textile, electromagnetically-acting stump liner: a randomized, double-blind, crossover study. J Pain Symptom Manage 2006; 32(4):352–60.

ELSEVIER
SAUNDERS

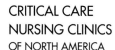

CRITICAL CARE
NURSING CLINICS
OF NORTH AMERICA

Crit Care Nurs Clin N Am 20 (2008) 59–65

# Nutrition Support of the Traumatically Injured Warfighter

Mary S. McCarthy, PhD, RN, CNSN[a],*,
Janet Fabling, RD, CNSD, CSP[a],
Robert Martindale, MD, PhD[b],
Stephanie Ann Meyer, MS, RD, MAJ, SP, USA[c]

[a]*Madigan Army Medical Center, ATTN: MCHJ-CON-NR, Tacoma, WA 98431, USA*
[b]*Oregon Health and Science University, 3181 SW Sam Jackson Park Rd. L223A, Portland, OR 97239, USA*
[c]*Medical Nutrition Therapy, Landstuhl Regional Medical Center, CMR 402,
Box 1591, APO, AE, 09180, Landstuhl, Germany*

Today's warfighters in Iraq are fighting a ground war against an adaptive enemy armed with highly lethal improvised explosive devices that can cause severe injuries requiring decisive interventions to save limbs and lives. Severe trauma leads to marked metabolic changes that disrupt cellular and systemic homeostasis. The hypermetabolism and hypercatabolism associated with neurotrauma, thermal injury, gunshot wounds, open fractures, and catastrophic amputations require early, aggressive nutritional therapy to restore cellular immune defenses and sustain vital organ functions in the face of extreme stress.

## Trauma on today's battlefield

According to hospital files, a wide variety of trauma-associated diagnoses were treated in the ICU at the theater evacuation hospital (the designated regional Army medical center that receives casualties) during a 1-year period. Of the trauma diagnoses, 19.5% were fractures,

16.6% were skull fractures, 16.2% were burns, 9% were amputations (all sites combined), 3% were intracranial injuries, and 1.5% were open head wounds. The remaining 34% of the wounded had experienced a variety of traumatic injuries including pneumothorax and hemothorax and open wounds of the eye, neck, chest, back, and lower torso. In addition, the files confirm crushing injuries, contusions, lacerations, sprains, and strains. (Authorized data retrieval by S. Meyer, May 2007). Patients with these types of traumatic injuries previously occupied theater ICU beds for prolonged periods of time but now are evacuated rapidly to definitive care outside the combat environment [1]. Although valuable lessons can be learned from the types of traumatic injuries sustained by warfighters on the modern battlefield, aggressive resuscitation, surgical stabilization, and early goal-directed metabolic therapies such as glycemic control and nutrition support are applicable to all victims of trauma.

This article presents the rationale for early nutritional support while sharing current evidence related to assessment, determination of energy expenditure, appropriate formula selection, and monitoring to prevent complications. Ideally, nutrition support of the critically wounded provides the nutrients necessary to balance hypermetabolic processes, heal wounds, and promote optimal recovery.

The views expressed in this manuscript are those of the authors and do not reflect the official policy of the Department of Army, Department of Defense, or US Government.

* Corresponding author.
*E-mail address:* mary.mccarthy@amedd.army.mil (M.S. McCarthy).

0899-5885/08/$ - see front matter. Published by Elsevier Inc.
doi:10.1016/j.ccell.2007.10.010

## Nutritional care

### Assessment of body composition

The patient's height and weight should be measured immediately. Body weight may fluctuate erratically following major trauma depending on the volume of resuscitation fluid required and the amount of time since resuscitation. There may be edema or ascites that can result in the retention of several liters of fluid, sometimes as much as 10 to 15 L. Additionally, malnutrition is associated with fluid shifts from the intravascular to extravascular space with a concurrent decline in lean body mass. Over time, loss of lean body mass often is masked, with little obvious change in body weight [2]. Dry weight and height are used to calculate the body mass index. Normal body mass index is considered to be 19 to 25 $kg/m^2$. Weight should be measured weekly, noting that acute weight changes are most likely caused by fluid shifts.

### Biochemical measurements

Evaluation of serum protein levels (eg, albumin and prealbumin) often is used to help assess the patient's nutritional status. These proteins have transport functions separate from their use in nutrition assessment, so they have variable sensitivity as predictors of nutritional status [3]. The release of proinflammatory cytokines during metabolic stress initiates acute-phase reactant synthesis (C-reactive protein, fibrinogen), and reduces transport protein synthesis (albumin, prealbumin) [4,5]. Initially low levels of serum proteins are more reflective of illness severity and inflammatory state than of nutritional status.

### Fluid requirements

The primary goal of administered fluids is to maintain adequate urinary output and serum electrolyte levels. Typically, fluid requirements for nonfebrile patients are 35 mL/kg/d. Insensible fluid losses increase dramatically with fever and burns. Many traumatically injured patients, however, are at risk for volume overload with large amounts of fluids administered for fluid resuscitation, antibiotics, and other medications.

### Energy and protein requirements

In the traumatically injured patient, the goals of nutrition support are to minimize the loss of body cell mass and to provide adequate nutrients to support wound healing, immune function, and hypermetabolism. Nutrition support should serve as an adjunct to other critical therapies. The early provision of nutrient substrates to support cellular processes can attenuate a portion of the protein loss but cannot reverse the acute catabolic influence of the traumatic injury [6]. Instituting early nutritional intervention will help achieve fluid balance, begin to restore body proteins, reduce infection risk by strengthening immune responses, and maintain critical organ functions.

One of the most important decisions in providing nutrition support to patients involves an accurate assessment of required calories. It has been demonstrated that traumatic injuries, specifically burns and head injuries, significantly accelerate the metabolic rate and therefore energy requirements [7,8]. In the case of severe traumatic brain injury (TBI), moderate to severe hypermetabolism may persist 4 to 6 weeks after injury [9]. In the first 2 weeks after injury, it is difficult to ascertain nutrition needs because the metabolic response overshadows developing nutritional deficiencies as fluid status, shock, and sepsis significantly affect laboratory values and body weight.

There are two methods for determining an individual's energy requirements: measurement of energy expenditure (indirect calorimetry), or the use of predictive equations. Portable indirect calorimeters provide the reference standard in measurement by quantifying oxygen consumption and carbon dioxide production over a 30-minute period. More commonly, clinicians use one of more than 200 predictive equations that have been developed for estimating energy expenditure. A consensus statement from the American College of Chest Physicians suggests that providing 25 kcal/kg of usual body weight is adequate for many patients in intensive care [3]. In TBI, however, the range of energy expenditure has been reported as 0.75 to 2.5 times normal. Nitrogen losses in TBI are similar to those in patients who have 20% to 40% body surface area burns with an average nitrogen excretion of 20 g/d during the acute-injury phase [10,11].

The hypermetabolism and catabolism in burn patients generally are directly proportional to the depth and size of the burn [12]. It is undisputed that energy and protein needs are heightened postburn and that adequate, but not excessive, calories should be provided [13]. Generally, burn formulas incorporate a factor of 20% to 30% above measured energy expenditure to account for increased calorie demands from physical therapy along with the stresses of wound care [12].

Although the optimal caloric load for the hypermetabolic surgical patient remains undetermined, the caloric delivery currently considered safe for the severely traumatized individual is in the range of 20 to 30 kcal/kg/d [14]. Protein delivery should remain at the level of 1.5 to 2.0 g /kg ideal body weight throughout the postinjury period because the protein needs of trauma patients are significantly increased compared with patients experiencing simple starvation [15]. Unfed TBI patients can lose up to 10% of lean body mass in a week, 25% in 2 weeks, and 30% to 40% in 3 weeks, which can increase morbidity and mortality [16]. Most studies examining protein intakes in septic, injured, or burned patients have found no benefit to giving protein in excess of 1.5 to 2 g/kg ideal body weight [11].

*Carbohydrate requirements*

The amount of carbohydrate provided should be the amount adequate to spare the use of protein for energy while also avoiding hyperglycemia. The minimum requirements have been estimated at 40% to 60% of total energy needs in critically ill patients; this level of intake is achieved using most standard nutritional formulas. Excessive carbohydrate calories as well as total calories can contribute to worsening hyperglycemia, especially for patients who are diabetics, receiving steroids, or who are experiencing stress-induced hyperglycemia. Although nutrition support should assist with ICU goals to maintain blood glucose at a safe level, intensive insulin therapy now is recognized as the preferred method to achieve optimal blood glucose control.

*Lipid requirements*

Most experts agree that 25% to 30% of total daily energy needs should be administered as fat, not exceeding 1 g/kg/d [17]. The omega-3 fats in fish oil (eicosapentaenoic acid, [EPA] and gamma-linolenic acid) have been shown to have multiple beneficial effects in trauma patients, including modulation of leukocyte function and regulation of cytokine release through nuclear signaling and gene expression [18,19]. The route of delivery of omega-3 fats also may be of importance. Using the enteral route, it takes at least 3 to 5 days to achieve adequate EPA levels in the plasma membrane to elicit the beneficial influence on the prostaglandin cascade. When omega-3 fats are given parenterally, however, a clinically relevant response can be achieved in as little as 3

hours [20,21]. Omega-3 fats are found in several immune-modulating formulas. Although the immune-modulating formulas containing omega-3 fats have not been adopted for all disease states manifesting an altered immunologic response, their use in trauma seems safe and appropriate to prevent late infectious complications. Omega-6 fats also should be administered periodically to prevent essential fatty acid deficiency (ie, at least 4% of total calories) [3].

*Micronutrient requirements*

Because protein and energy needs usually increase with traumatic injury, it is assumed that micronutrient requirements must be increased as well, even though no specific requirements are known at this time. Enrichment of vitamins A (5000 IU/1000 kcal) and C (500 mg twice daily) and zinc sulfate (200 mg daily) or elemental zinc (50 mg daily) is indicated in large burns [22]. The trace element deficiencies associated with burns are attributed to extensive cutaneous exudative losses and, to a lesser extent, urinary losses, drains, and hemorrhage, which cause negative micronutrient balances during the first week after injury. Copper deficiency is specific to burns. Warfighters can lose 20% to 40% of their body copper stores within the first week of injury when the burn wound involves 20% or more of the total body surface area. Plasma copper concentrations can remain low for weeks; they will be proportional to the burn size and may cause fatal arrhythmias [22]. Daily zinc supplementation (10–12 mg) is recommended in the head-injured patient [23]. Excess urinary zinc is associated with hypermetabolism, poor wound healing, and depressed immune function [24].

*Selecting the appropriate route for feeding*

There is consensus among trauma surgeons and intensive care physicians that early enteral feeding is the preferred route for nutrition support, but before initiating enteral feeding the end points of shock resuscitation must be achieved. The enteral route is associated with significantly fewer septic complications than total parenteral nutrition [25]. The enteral route also is favored because of its demonstrated ability to blunt the hypermetabolic response, support the gut-associated lymphoid tissue, increase visceral protein synthesis [26], and limit cost [27]. Burn patients, in particular, who are fed enterally within 24 hours of injury show less endotoxin absorption from the gut than patients who are fed after 48 hours [28]. Although there may be additional benefits to metabolically stressed patients, the major advantage of enteral over parenteral nutrition has been manifested in improved clinical outcomes with increased survival rates and reduced morbidity, specifically infectious complications [26]. The latest reports from United States military hospitals in Germany indicate that the majority of injured warfighters are being fed into the jejunum so that feedings can continue during procedures in the operating room and during the transport back to the United States. (S. Meyer, personal communication, February 2007)

*Formula selection—enteral*

Although high-protein enteral formulas may be adequate for most trauma patients, the best evidence available today suggests that immune-modulating formulas are superior to standard formulas because of their ability to improve clinically important outcomes in patients sustaining the most severe injuries from trauma. Results of the 34 currently published peer reviewed studies suggest that immune-modulating formulas containing omega-3 fatty acids, glutamine, arginine, RNA nucleotides, and antioxidant vitamins A, C, and E offer a benefit to certain patient populations in terms of reduced rates of infection, decreased antibiotic use, lowered incidence of intra-abdominal abscesses, and reduced ICU and hospital length of stay [29]. The populations most likely to benefit include patients who will undergo complicated gastrointestinal surgery, who have sustained severe trauma, or have experienced a complicated ICU stay.

An immune-modulating formula currently being used by clinicians treating wounded warfighters in Germany is high in protein, and contains omega-3 fatty acids, glutamine, arginine, and dietary nucleotides; it also contains 10 g of fiber per liter and antioxidant vitamins A, C, and E (S. Meyer, personal communication, February 1, 2007). Multicenter prospective, randomized clinical trials in critically ill trauma patients have demonstrated that the administration of an immune-modulating formula for 7 to 10 days reduced the rates of infection, wound complications, and the risk of multiple organ failure [29,30].

For patients who do not tolerate an immune-modulating formula or who are septic, a fiber-fortified, isotonic formula that is moderate in protein can be used. For the young, traumatically injured warfighter, additional protein and glutamine is usually provided. Trauma patients generally receive up to 30 g of glutamine enterally each day.

Elemental or predigested formulas also have been developed for conditions of stress, trauma, and malabsorption. These formulas are moderate in protein and contain omega-3 fatty acids and arginine. Unique to this type of formula is the inclusion of fructo-oligosaccharides, which are natural carbohydrates that are not digested in the gastrointestinal tract but are fermented to short-chain fatty acids by gram-negative organisms such as bifidobacteria in the colon. Short-chain fatty acids are the preferred fuel of the cells of the colon and help maintain gut mucosal integrity. The fructo-oligosaccharides are classified as dietary fiber but do not contribute to residue in the stool. They are referred to as "prebiotics" because they stimulate the growth of healthy intestinal bacteria [31].

*Formula selection—parenteral*

Parenteral nutrition was developed primarily to provide nutrition to those unable to take adequate nutrition through the gastrointestinal tract because of the loss of absorptive surface and/or the inability to ingest or digest nutrients. A nonfunctioning gastrointestinal tract and/or failure to tolerate enteral nutrition remain the primary indications for parenteral nutrition. Although parenteral nutrition can be lifesaving when used appropriately, it can result in numerous adverse clinical outcomes. The gastrointestinal tract functions not only to digest and absorb nutrients; it also is the body's largest immunologic organ. Approximately 60% of the body's immunoglobulin-producing cells line the gastrointestinal tract, and 80% of the body's manufactured immunoglobulin is secreted across the gastrointestinal mucosa [32]. During major traumatic injury, a relative or absolute gut ischemia can occur, leading to mucosal compromise, disruption of the gut's barrier function, and ultimately passage of bacteria and toxins into the bloodstream or mesenteric lymphoid system. In addition, common clinical practices such as the use of broad-spectrum antibiotics, proton-pump inhibitors, $H_2$ blockers, and narcotics, as well as physiologic and inflammatory changes during acute stress, can lead to gastrointestinal dysmotility and bacterial overgrowth in the proximal gastrointestinal tract, impacting the gut's protective barrier [33]. Animal studies clearly show that enteral rather than parenteral nutrition maintains gut integrity and immune responsiveness and prevents bacterial translocation [33–35].

Carbohydrate is the primary energy source in parenteral solutions. It is estimated that a minimum of 100 g of glucose is needed for tissues with an obligate glucose requirement such as the central nervous system, white blood cells, red blood cells, and renal medulla. Each gram of dextrose provides 3.4 kcal. The patient's carbohydrate requirements can be calculated as 40% to 60% of total daily calories. The guideline for parenteral protein (1.5–2.0 g/kg/d) is the same as for oral/enteral formulas. Because of the adverse effects identified, it now is recommended that lipid administration be limited to 1 g/kg/d or 25% to 30% of total calories. In patients who have severe infections or sepsis, intravenous lipids should be given only in the amount necessary to meet essential fatty acid needs [17].

*Monitoring nutrition support*

Although much emphasis is placed on early initiation of nutrition support in the trauma patient, it is equally important to monitor the enteral and/or parenteral regimen. Underfeeding of both calories and protein related to gut dysfunction and interruption for procedures is common. On average, patients receive 75% of the amount of feeding prescribed [36,37]. Metabolic derangements, such as changes in phosphorus, potassium, magnesium, and glucose metabolism as well as the need for fluid resuscitation may all be present in the trauma patient. The direction of trends in serum protein levels, not individual values, should be used to determine the adequacy of protein intake. When a positive trend is not observed, monitoring an acute-phase reactant (eg, C-reactive protein) along with a short-turnover protein (eg, prealbumin) may be helpful. As the inflammatory process is resolving, acute-phase reactants should decrease, and serum protein levels should increase if nutrition is adequate. Overfeeding may contribute to hypercapnia, hyperglycemia, hypertriglyceridemia, hepatic steatosis, and myriad adverse metabolic side effects [14,38–40].

Other indices to monitor when determining adequacy of the nutrition support regimen include the rate of wound healing, the patient's functional status, ability to tolerate ventilator-weaning strategies, and overall stamina to work with other therapies, such as physical and speech therapy.

Although enteral feeding is preferred to intravenous or parenteral feeding in trauma, patients sometimes do not tolerate it. A patient who has TBI and a low Glasgow Coma Scale score (3–8) tends to have a more prolonged gastric ileus and will be less likely to tolerate enteral feedings immediately after injury [41]. Signs of intolerance include abdominal distension, formula reflux, increased gastric residuals, nausea, vomiting, diarrhea, and abdominal pain. If intolerance of enteral nutrition continues for more than 72 hours, parenteral feeding should be considered. A preponderance of data suggests that enteral feeding below the pylorus and before bowel sounds are heard is usually tolerated and helps preserve intestinal mucosa integrity. The risk for aspiration exists to some extent in all tube-fed patients, depending on gastrointestinal dysmotility patterns and individual patient characteristics. One of the most important assessment parameters to monitor is gastric emptying, best measured at the bedside using the gastric residual volume (GRV). An excessive GRV predisposes the patient to gastroesophageal reflux and aspiration; therefore, if a high GRV can be detected early, aspiration may be prevented. The critical level of GRV is not known, but recommendations are that GRVs, initially measured every 4 to 6 hours in the range of 200 to 500 mL should prompt careful bedside evaluation, and GRVs greater than 500 mL warrant withholding of feedings and reassessment of the patient's tolerance of tube feeding. Other measures that can be taken to reduce the risk of aspiration include elevating the head of the bed to more than 30° to 45°, the use of prokinetic agents, placing the feeding tube distal to the stomach and optimally beyond the ligament of Treitz, reassessing need, level, and choice of agents for sedation, and considering continuous aspiration of subglottic secretions [42].

**Summary**

Four signature injuries have been associated with the current conflict: TBI, posttraumatic stress disorder, increased survival after severe burns, and traumatic amputations. The combined impact of the severe metabolic derangements in trauma, including hypermetabolism, hyperglycemia with insulin resistance, and net protein catabolism, along with bed rest, inactivity, and lack of nutritional intake can lead to rapid and significant depletion of lean body mass. Nutrition support cannot fully prevent or reverse the metabolic alterations and disruptions in body composition associated with critical illness; it is supportive, in that it can slow the rate of net protein catabolism. Nutrition support can be thought of as a therapy for "metabolic resuscitation" [43] that requires the formula selection to be tailored to maintain integrity of the gut barrier and function, to reduce regional oxidative stress, and to modify or perhaps augment cellular immune functions. Maintenance of host immunity is still the best defense to reduce infectious complications and mortality. There is agreement that provision of 1.5 to 2.0 g/kg/d of protein is sufficient to minimize losses of body protein during the initial 2 weeks of trauma or critical illness. Information is lacking regarding requirements for minerals, vitamins, and trace elements during critical illness. Armed with current scientific knowledge, nutritional support of the traumatically injured warfighter should be approached early, aggressively, and with the understanding that safe, well-tolerated nutrition is the optimal strategy to ensure the best short- and long-term clinical outcomes.

# References

[1] Earwood J, Brooks D. The seven P's in battalion level combat health support in the Military Operations in Urban Terrain environment: the Fallujah experience, summer 2003 to spring 2004. Mil Med 2006;171(4):273–7.

[2] Hammond D. History and physical examination. In: Matarese L, Gottschlich M, editors. Contemporary nutrition support practice. Philadelphia: WB Saunders Co; 1998. p. 25–6.

[3] Cerra F, Benitez M, Blackburn G, et al. Applied nutrition in ICU patients: a consensus statement of the American College of Chest Physicians. Chest 1997; 111:769–78.

[4] Martindale R, Shikora S, Nishikawa R, et al. The metabolic response to stress and alterations in nutrient metabolism. In: Shikora S, Martindale R, editors. Nutritional considerations in the intensive care unit. Iowa: Kendall Hunt; 2002. p. 11–21.

[5] Plank L, Hill G. Sequential metabolic changes following induction of systemic inflammatory response in patients with severe sepsis and major blunt trauma. World J Surg 2000;24:630–8.

[6] Frankenfield D, Smith J, Cooney R. Accelerated nitrogen loss after traumatic injury is not attenuated by achievement of energy balance. JPEN J Parenter Enteral Nutr 1997;21:324–9.

[7] Turner JW, Ireton C, Hunt J, et al. Predicting energy expenditures in burned patients. J Trauma 1985;25: 11–7.

[8] Long C, Schaffel N, Geiger J, et al. Metabolic response to injury and illness: estimation of energy and protein needs form indirect calorimetry and nitrogen balance. JPEN J Parenter Enteral Nutr 1979;3:452–9.

[9] Young B, Ott L, Norton J, et al. Metabolic and nutritional sequelae in the non-steroid treated head injury patient. Neurosurgery 1985;17(5): 784–91.

[10] Clifton G, Robertson C, Grossman R, et al. The metabolic response to severe head injury. J Neurosurg 1984;60(4):687–96.

[11] A.S.P.E.N. Guidelines for the use of parenteral and enteral nutrition in adult and pediatric patients. JPEN J Parenter Enteral Nutr 2002;17(Suppl): 20SA–1SA.

[12] Mayes T, Gottschlich M. Burns and wound healing. In: Gottschlich M, editor. The science and practice of nutrition support. A case-based core curriculum. Dubuque (IN): Kendall Hunt Publishing Co.; 2001. p. 391–420.

[13] Peck M. American Burn Association clinical guidelines: initial support of burn patients. J Burn Care Rehabil 2001;22:595–665.

[14] Streat S, Beddoe A, Hill G. Aggressive nutritional support does not prevent protein loss despite fat gain in septic intensive care patients. J Trauma 1987;27:262–6.

[15] Briet F, Jeejeebhoy K. Effect of hypoenergetic feeding and refeeding on muscle and mononuclear cell activities of mitochondrial complexes I-IV in enterally fed rats. Am J Clin Nutr 2001;73:975–83.

[16] Hadley M. Nutrition support of head-injured patients. Int J Appl Basic Sci 1996;12:126–7.

[17] Hasselmann M, Reimund J. Lipids in nutritional support of critically ill patients. Curr Opin Crit Care 2004;10:449–55.

[18] Calder P, Grimble R. Polyunsaturated fatty acids, inflammation and immunity. Eur J Clin Nutr 2002; 56:S14–9.

[19] Sweeney B, Puri P, Reen D. Modulation of immune cell function by polyunsaturated fatty acids. Pediatr Surg Int 2005;21:335–40.

[20] Roy C, Bouthillier L, Seidman E, et al. New lipids in enteral feeding. Curr Opin Clin Nutr Metab Care 2004;7:117–22.

[21] Mayer K, Gokorsch S, Fegbeutel C, et al. Parenteral nutrition with fish oil modulates cytokine response in patients with sepsis. Am J Respir Crit Care Med 2003;167:1321–8.

[22] Gamliel Z, DeBiasse M, Demling R. Essential microminerals and their response to burn injury. J Burn Care Rehabil 1996;17(3):264–72.

[23] Samuels M, editor. Manual of neurologic therapeutics and essentials of diagnosis. 3rd edition. Boston: Little, Brown; 1986.

[24] McClain C, Henning B, Ott L, et al. Mechanisms and implications of hypoalbuminemia in head-injured patients. J Neurosurg 1988;69(3):386–92.

[25] Moore F, Moore E, Jones T, et al. TEN versus TPN following major abdominal trauma: reduced septic morbidity. J Trauma 1989;29:916–23.

[26] Suchner U, Senftleben U, Eckart T, et al. Enteral vs parenteral nutrition: effects on gastrointestinal function and metabolism. Nutrition 1996;12(1):13–22.

[27] Braga M, Gianotti L, Gentilini P, et al. Early postoperative enteral nutrition improves gut oxygenation and reduces cost compared with total parenteral nutrition. Crit Care Med 2001;29:242–8.

[28] Peng Y, Yuan Z, Xiao G. Effects of enteral feeding on the prevention of enterogenic infection in severely burned patients. Burns 2001;27:145–9.

[29] Proceedings from the Summit on Immune-Enhancing Enteral Therapy May 25–26, 2000. JPEN J Parenter Enteral Nutr 2001;25:S1–63.

[30] Montejo J, Zarazaga A, Lopez-Martinez J, et al. Immunonutrition in the intensive care unit. A systematic review and consensus statement. Clin Nutr 2003;22:221–3.

[31] Ross (Nutrition) 2006 pocket guide. Ohio: Ross Products Division, Abbott Laboratories, Inc.; 2006.

[32] King B, Kudsk K, Li J, et al. Route and type of nutrition influence mucosal immunity to bacterial pneumonia. Ann Surg 1999;229:272–8.

[33] Kotani J, Usami M, Nomura H, et al. Enteral nutrition prevents bacterial translocation but does not improve survival during acute pancreatitis. Arch Surg 1999;134:287–92.

[34] King B, Li J, Kudsk K. A temporal study of TPN-induced changes in gut-associated lymphoid tissue and mucosal immunity. Arch Surg 1997;132:1303–9.

[35] Li J, Kudsk K, Gocinski B, et al. Effects of parenteral and enteral nutrition on gut-associated lymphoid tissue. J Trauma 1995;39:44–51.

[36] Kozar R, McQuiggan M, Moore E, et al. Postinjury enteral tolerance is reliably achieved by a standardized protocol. J Surg Res 2002;104:70–5.

[37] DeJonghe B, Appere-De-Vechi C, Fournier M, et al. A prospective survey of nutritional support practices in intensive care unit patients: what is prescribed? What is delivered? Crit Care Med 2001;29:8–12.

[38] Shaw J, Wildbore M, Wolfe R. Whole body protein kinetics in severely septic patients. Ann Surg 1987;205:288–94.

[39] Pomposelli J, Baxter J, Babineau T, et al. Early postoperative glucose control predicts nosocomial infection rate in diabetic patients. JPEN J Parenter Enteral Nutr 1998;22:77–81.

[40] Dahn M, Mitchell R, Lange M, et al. Hepatic metabolic response to injury and sepsis. Surgery 1995;117:520–30.

[41] Evans N, Compher C. Nutrition and the neurologically impaired patient. In: Torosian M, editor. Nutrition for the hospitalized patient. New York: Marcel Dekker; 1995. p. 567–90.

[42] McClave S, DeMeo M, DeLegge M, et al. North American Summit on Aspiration in the Critically Ill Patient: consensus statement. JPEN J Parenter Enteral Nutr 2002;26(Suppl 6):S80–5.

[43] Heyland D, Dhaliwal R. Oxidative stress in the critically ill: a preliminary look at the REDOXS study. Critical Care Rounds 2006;7(1):1–6.

ELSEVIER
SAUNDERS

Crit Care Nurs Clin N Am 20 (2008) 67–71

CRITICAL CARE
NURSING CLINICS
OF NORTH AMERICA

# Memories of Three Wars: A Nurse's Story

## Loretta J. Aiken, RN, MSN*

*National Naval Medical Center, 8901 Wisconsin Avenue, Bethesda, MD 20889, USA*

War! Just hearing that one little word can bring flashes of memory and a cold chill to my body. It makes my mind wander back over my long nursing career and the three generations of American warfighters I have worked with who suffered physical and emotional trauma from their war injuries. It also brings back some of my dearest memories as a nurse and the pure joy of knowing I helped make a difference in their lives.

I think about working for the Veterans Administration during the Vietnam era and all the young veterans I met then. Some had gunshot wounds, some had emotional wounds, and some could not cope with how their country felt about the unpopular war. As a nurse, I was an eyewitness to the personal and emotional struggles young soldiers faced on their long roads to recovery. Many suffered severely debilitating combat injuries, others had lingering infections picked up in a distant land, and yet others had no outward injuries but wrestled with demons of drugs or drink to forget their war experiences. A few were bitter and reluctant to talk; others told unbelievably graphic stories about being under fire. Some gave first-hand accounts of the cruelties of war, and others had horrible flashbacks and nightmares of events suffered in battle.

Some of the veterans would not look at their wounds or discuss their future. Others cried about lost loves and how their young wives or girlfriends might never accept them again. All the young men were scarred in some personal way from their sacrifices for their country, and each one was

trying to return to a mainstream culture that might not accept his physical limitations. It was heart wrenching to see them trying to attain normal lives, but their personal courage and stamina were astonishing to me.

I remember one young soldier who had been especially close to my heart. I watched him try to convince himself he did not need his legs as long as he had his mind. We cried together during some of those long night shifts when I changed his dressings and gave him antibiotics. He was sure he would never marry or have a child, but he thought he might be good at teaching. I was sick at heart for his loss and knew how deeply he had been affected by the land mine he had stepped on. I couldn't imagine life without my own legs, and I was awed by his stamina and determination. His life had been changed forever in 1 second, but it had taken him 2 years to accept his injuries and his fate. Life had dealt him a terrible blow, but somehow he managed to overcome his loss. The last time I heard from him, he was well into a doctoral program at a large university in the Midwest and had just married his laboratory partner.

Throughout their stays on my ward, we laughed and joked together and formed the bonds I remember to this day. I will never forget the fun we had under such bad circumstances, and I loved the way the patients genuinely cared for each other. I was in my early twenties, but I was still older than most of the young veterans. It was a rare night that I didn't get a marriage proposal or pledge of undying love, but it was all in light-hearted fun to help them pass the lonely times away from their loved ones. It was also a test for them to learn to laugh and flirt with someone their own age again.

The strong helped the weak, and they all looked out for each other. I was amazed how the older veterans from World War II and the Korean War gave words of encouragement and

The views expressed in this article are those of the author's and do not reflect the official policy of the Department of the Navy, the Department of Defense, nor the United States Government.

* 1605 South Barton Street, Arlington, VA 22204.

*E-mail address:* Loretta.Aiken@med.navy.mil

0899-5885/08/$ - see front matter. Published by Elsevier Inc.
doi:10.1016/j.ccell.2007.10.001

*ccnursing.theclinics.com*

pep talks to the younger veterans when times were hard. The older men assured the younger veterans that girls would still like them, and if all else failed in the romance department, they could just to pick an ugly girl who could cook. I still laugh when I think of all the talk about the importance of good cooking. It was a camaraderie I had never experienced before but have seen over and over again in veterans since then.

Preacher was my favorite patient from that era. He was from Alabama and had been shot in the leg while crawling through a rice paddy. Somehow he found the inner strength to keep a positive and upbeat spirit through his multiple surgeries and months of hospital stay. He told me dozens of times that his life had been saved for a reason, and he thought it was because he had been "called" to preach the gospel. I dreaded his nightly dressing changes, but Preacher had a way about him that put me at ease. He always sang old hymns or gospel songs to me while I worked, and he could make my most dreaded tasks seem like fun. I still remember those hymns and how sometimes other veterans in the eight-bed room would sing along with him in the wee hours of the night. To this day, I never hear "Amazing Grace" without thinking of Preacher so many years ago.

I still smile when I remember Preacher's excitement about dedicating his life to Christ and working to save lost souls. He had dreams of tent meetings and revivals in the rural South, and I lost track of the number of times he practiced sermons on me. His ability to say the right words at the right time helped his roommates cope with their own struggles and seemed to comfort me with my own work. We all teased him about how the church ladies would flock around him and whisper about his war injury. He told me over and over again about God's plan for him and how his war injury had been God's will.

I still get teary-eyed when I remember the day Preacher was discharged from the Veterans Administration hospital and how he gave me a bouquet of pink sweetheart roses and blew me a kiss. He was off to enjoy his life and to preach the Word. He had a new leg, a strong faith, and an old girlfriend who had been sending him love letters. His parting words to me were "Life can't get no better than this." I heard him humming as he walked down the hallway, and I knew in my heart he would do well. Those church ladies in Alabama really would dote on him, and he really would save lost souls and help people find new meaning to life.

I have thought of Preacher a million times over the years and still think of him as I work with young veterans of the current war who are trying just as desperately to adjust to loss of limbs and body image. He will never know how much I admired his courage and sense of humor, or what he taught me about the human suffering of war. He and I were from different backgrounds, different races, and different parts of the country, but my job as a nurse and his war injury put us in the same place at the same time. I have always thought that maybe Preacher's war injury was God's will for me also.

Many veterans I worked with over the years did not fare as well. Some were never able to accept their injuries, and many spiraled into lives of alcoholism, drug addiction, and violent behavior. Many veterans ended up alienated from their family members, and sometimes I would see homeless veterans on the streets. Once I ran in to one of my former patients sitting in a wheelchair near the Smithsonian Institution. I bought hot dogs and sodas for him and his buddies, and we had a wonderful picnic. They all said they just did not fit in normal society after the war and were happier on the streets. He laughed when I gave him a goodbye hug, and then he told me not to get too close. He said he had some bugs he needed to get rid of and was planning on a hot bath at the Gospel Mission. I itched all the way home, but I still treasured the memory of that chance encounter.

Viet Nam was just a distant memory for me in 1990 when I left the Veterans Administration hospital and went to work at the National Naval Medical Center (NNMC) in Bethesda, Maryland. Within only 2 short months, however, there was talk of war and preliminary plans for deployment of troops to the Persian Gulf. Suddenly, the United States was preparing for war, and I was back to thinking about land mines and paralyzed veterans and was recalling the years of pain and suffering I had witnessed after the last unpopular war.

I remember the President preparing the country for war and how the military prepared at the Naval Hospital. We trained for battle causalities, burns, bioterrorism, and massive body injuries. When the Navy active duty staff deployed for Desert Storm, reservists came in to "back-fill" the hospital with nursing and medical staff, so that the normal day-to-day operations could continue. We pulled together, watched the progress of the war on television, and waited for the wounded to arrive. We lived through the media blitzes, the popularity of the commanding generals, and the good wishes of a country that supported the war effort. "God Bless the USA" was on every radio station, and I remember it blaring through the loudspeakers in the shopping malls and grocery stores.

We waited for the war to start and for the injured to arrive. Finally, on the appointed night, we watched in absolute amazement as the war unfolded on the small television screen that we pulled into the nurses' lounge. We saw air attacks, smart bombs, and explosions as we ate dinner, and each of us mentally clicked off the time before the injured would arrive. Within the next 2 weeks, a few casualties did arrive, but certainly not as many as we expected. We had new technologies, new antibiotics, and new treatment modalities that were far more sophisticated than during the Viet Nam War. Our rehabilitation capabilities were better, and many advances had been made in the field of surgery and prosthetics. I was 20 years older for the Desert Storm War than I had been for the Viet Nam War, and I had 20 more years of experience as an ICU nurse. Then, just as we were really gearing up to accept incoming wounded, the Desert Storm War was over, and we were told the troops would be coming home. Even though my second war had not been as bad as the first, it took a toll on all of us and made each of us wonder just how long it might be until the next one.

After September 11, 2001, I knew for the third time in my nursing career that I would be called to help my country through another war. The talk of war made me think of all of my travels as a tourist throughout the Middle East and the wonderful people who had been so nice to me. I remembered the delicious food, the happy children, and the exotic beauty of countries so different from my own. I also remembered the poverty, the lack of resources, and all the people who faced the hardships of living in Third World nations. I thought about the treasured items I had purchased in small village markets and my memories of Arab women and children in everyday activities of life. Some of these people seemed to have so little, and I worried that what little they had might be taken away.

I thought of my own fears and how I would react to another generation of young men with amputations, severed spines, and blast wounds. I thought of parents sending sons and daughters off to war, and I prayed that I had taught the medical corpsmen enough to survive on the battlefield. I thought of the junior staff who worked with me and how they would react to the horrors of wounds, burns, and explosive injuries. The thoughts of this war affected me more than the other two wars, perhaps because of my age and the thoughts of history repeating itself. I had spent more than 30 years of my life as a nurse, and I hoped I was prepared for what the coming months would bring.

Several hundred NNMC staff members deployed to the USNS Comfort, which is one of the two hospital ships of the Navy, during the first week of March in 2003. We all knew we had reached the point of no political return, and everyone predicted the war would start within a week. The country was at the highest terrorism alert level, and the local communities were preparing for a potential catastrophic event. We talked nonstop of war injuries, smallpox, anthrax, dirty bombs, and fatal gas attacks in the subways and shopping malls. I lived within a mile of the Pentagon and took every threat very seriously. We had no idea what would occur during the coming months, but we were as prepared as possible for any event. The World Trade Center and Pentagon tragedies had taught us well, and no one minimized the impact that the looming war would have on the country.

Finally, on a fateful Wednesday in the third week of March 2003 an ultimatum was set, and a line was drawn. I thought of the corpsmen and medics on the front lines, and I thought of the fear the soldiers must be experiencing at the thought of the war starting. I thought of their parents who were waiting, just like me. I dreaded turning on my television but could not bring myself to ignore the news. The deadline was set at 8 PM, and we all knew President Bush would not back down. A few minutes after 8 PM, I heard an announcement that explosions had been heard in Baghdad. I hoped that 33 years of critical care nursing had prepared me for what I would be facing during the next few months or few years.

The next week was truly an awesome time to be working at NNMC. The whole staff pulled together, and we knew we could depend on each other. As the casualties started to come in, we had the experience and ability to deal with what arrived with each new planeload of medical evacuations. The shock and horror of the injuries were just as sickening to me as they had been so many years before, but I was astounded at the survival rates. I think I had never truly grasped the concept of modern medicine until I saw the battle injuries and how far medicine had progressed during the last 30 years.

The people of America really did rally behind the troops again this time, and the dignitaries and famous people that came to visit the wounded were very impressive. Members of Congress, movie stars, beauty queens, cheerleaders, and sports figures came to visit and give words of support. Purple Hearts were given out to casualties in ceremonies in the ICU, and the patients' families became our own families. We hugged each other, cried together, and rejoiced at the advances of the young men who had been so gravely injured.

I told my Viet Nam tales to the wounded patients and assured them they would get better in time. Once again, one particular young patient touched my heart. I realized he could easily have been my child lying in the bed, so gravely injured and horribly disfigured. As I brushed his teeth and shaved him, I talked to him about some of my previous disabled veterans who had gone on to lead normal lives and do great deeds.

One patient, with multiple amputations, had become a well-known politician; another was a best-selling author who wrote of his land mine injuries. I told him about the brotherhood of the Paralyzed Veterans Association and how he would go to rehabilitation and learn to accept his own personal destiny of life in a wheelchair. He looked to me for assurance and guidance and asked me many times what he could do with the rest of his life. I told him he could teach, he could write, he could talk, and most of all he could love. I told him his life was not over and assured him he would find his way to joy and happiness again.

And then I went home and cried. I cried for the beautiful young body that was so grotesquely mangled and scarred. I cried for this young man who had joined the Marines so proud and fit, and with such great dreams of the glory of battle, who would never walk again. I cried because his entire life had changed within a fraction of a second, and I cried for his mother, I cried for his father, and I cried for the long uphill road he faced before he could ever have life of any normalcy.

Finally I cried for the entire country, and all the pain and suffering another war had brought to another generation of American youth. I cried all evening and the next morning on the way to work, and then I stopped crying. It was time to go back to the ICU and to take my place beside the others who were doing just what I had been doing for so many years.

In early May 2003, the President gave a speech, and I thought it meant we had won the war. My thoughts ran back over the last few months—the ups and downs and all the things that had happened from the beginning of the year. I thought of the long work hours, the emotional turmoil, the fear, the anxiety, and, most of all, the lives that would be forever affected by just a few weeks in March and April of 2003. I thought of young soldiers in the field who were scarred for life by being in battle for the first time. I thought of funerals, and flag ceremonies, and children who would never see their mothers or fathers again. I thought of the USNS Comfort staff who had so nobly left their family and friends behind and gone off to war. I thought of the group of reservists who had merged so quickly with the civilian nurses, and how we had become such a strong and united front to fill our mission at NNMC. Most of all, I thought about everything I had learned about myself and my abilities in my third war as a critical care nurse.

I thought of all of us on the home front who had put aside personal fears and had come together as a group with a goal on which our fighting force depended. No acts of terrorism had happened at home, but we knew we could have handled them if they had occurred. We had not let our troops down, and we had not let ourselves down. The antiwar protestors had not become violent, and we were all thankful that we lived in a country of free speech and free will, which allowed its citizens to express their own feelings about national concerns. I thought of the many leaders of this country who had been so personally affected by the war. I thought of the media and the veterans of previous wars who had been so supportive of the troops during this war and hoped the people of Iraq really would find the peace, health, and freedom that we so desperately wished for them. Most of all, I thought the war was over.

It is now more than 4 years later, and the medical evacuation planes still arrive on a regular basis from Germany. It is also a rare day that the *Washington Post* does not run a story about a marine's, sailor's, airman's, or soldier's life and funeral. I have witnessed injuries that the medical personnel thought the patient could not survive, but some of these young men have come back a year later to thank us for saving their lives. I have seen the most anguished deaths of my career, and I once spent an entire day on a crying binge when a marine sent me a picture of himself dressed in his uniform. I saw the handsome young man and could barely recognize him as the young bridegroom who had lost both legs and his eye from a blast injury. His shattered face and missing limbs had haunted me until I saw for myself how all our efforts had put him back together again. I'll always remember the weeks he spent in our ICU and how his father stood at the foot of his bed every evening and prayed he would live through the night. Somehow, just looking at the picture seemed to put my life in focus and made me remember the awesome teamwork that gave this young man back his life.

I daily ask myself how we have coped with the war and our losses and wonder how we manage to continue to do what we have done for so long. Sadly, I have no hope the war will end any time soon. This war has left its mark on me as well as the families of the dead and wounded. In August, 2007, I started my thirty-eighth year as a critical care nurse. My third war has been no easier than the others, but I have learned immensely from this experience. Sometimes I think of centuries of war and about the nurses throughout the ages who have cared for the battlefield wounded. The conflicts are different, and different groups of people are fighting under a different set of circumstances, but war is war, and history really does seem to repeat itself. As with all experiences, however, many good times come from the worst of times. War brings pain and suffering, the most unimaginable physical struggles, and death, but it also brings hope, faith, brotherhood, and human kindness.

As I have reflected over the last three wars, I can't believe that the time has gone by so quickly. I cherish my memories of patients, and sometimes, out of the blue, I think of one of the wounded veterans who has left such a mark on me. It still makes me very happy when marines, sailors, airmen, and soldiers come back to visit and ask for me. I see their mothers and fathers in the hospital cafeteria, and we hug each other like long-lost friends. I think of commanding generals and admirals shedding tears at Purple Heart ceremonies, and I watch the faces of young men who are missing eyes and limbs who come back to give words of encouragement to their buddies who are not so lucky. I see the emotional drain on families and watch tense family relationships sometimes deteriorate into open hostilities in the waiting room. I see the bonds of a mother's love, and I know how battle injuries can reunite broken families. I have watched young wives with babies on their hips and wondered in awe at how they cope with the strain and stress; they are so strong in their belief that all will get better. I grieved over the death of a young marine, and witnessed the total inconsolableness of the doctors, nurses, and every one else who had worked so desperately to save him. I also see the triumph of the human spirit in these young marines when they tell me they are eager to get a new arm, leg, or eye and go back to Iraq or Afghanistan to serve with their unit.

My experiences through these last three wars have been incredible. I have increased my own knowledge of trauma and surgeries, amputations, infections, head injuries, and human emotion by 100-fold . I hope that I have imparted some of my knowledge to the younger nurses, corpsmen, and ancillary staff who have worked with me and who will carry on the nursing profession long after I have retired. I enjoy my job as a nurse more than ever, and even though I do not bend in the places I did nearly 40 years ago, I am still strong and am involved with the profession to which I have dedicated my entire working life.

A few months ago, I was gently reminded of my age when I was working with a young marine in the ICU. I smiled when he told me he liked me because I reminded him of his mother's mother. I held his hand and told him that nothing could make me happier than to be compared with someone he loved so much. That incident reminded me that my life as a nurse has gone full circle. I am no longer the popular young nurse with all the marriage proposals. Instead I am the grandmother figure who teases them about finding a wife who can cook.

ELSEVIER
SAUNDERS

Crit Care Nurs Clin N Am 20 (2008) 73–81

CRITICAL CARE
NURSING CLINICS
OF NORTH AMERICA

# PTSD: Therapeutic Interventions Post-Katrina

Jacqueline Rhoads, PhD, APRN, ACNP-BC, ANP-C, CCRN, FAANP[a,*],
Timothy Pearman, PhD[b], Susan Rick, DNS, APRN[a]

[a]LSUHSC School of Nursing, 1900 Gravier Street, New Orleans, LA 70112, USA
[b]Tulane University Medical Center, Tulane Avenue, New Orleans, LA 70112, USA

I saw people lying all over the ground sick, tired and mentally exhausted. People of all ages who had collapsed from the heat and lack of water. A steady flow of elderly, some complaining of chest pain and others with shortness of breath all streaming across the bridge because it was the highest place free of water and where they hoped to be evacuated. How they got there only God knows. All looking to us to help get them to safety. We had little equipment and a few oxygen tanks—we had to ration what we had... clean out $O_2$ masks and then give the oxygen to those who needed it the most.... five minutes for each... [Health care provider personal account, September, 2007.]

August 29, 2006, brought the largest, most deadly hurricane ever to strike the Gulf Coast. According to reports, the storm killed more than 2000 people and destroyed billions of dollars of property with winds clocked at 160 to 175 mph [1]. More than a million residents were displaced, many requiring care for chronic conditions who suddenly also needed care for acute stress symptoms [2]. Today, many individuals still struggle to cope with major psychiatric posttraumatic stress disorders (PTSD). Using a case study approach, this article discusses PTSD, including what it is, how it manifests, how to diagnose it, patient education, and how it can be managed with therapeutic interventions. Special circumstances related to children are briefly presented.

Paul is a 46-year-old paramedic who presented to a mental health clinic in New Orleans, Louisiana complaining of insomnia. He states he has had this difficulty for the past year and feels it is related to his experiences as a search and rescue paramedic after Hurricane Katrina. He has been a veteran of the New Orleans Search and Rescue Squad for 16 years and is well liked by his peers. He is married, but after the storm his wife wanted to remain in Houston with her family and he refused to leave New Orleans, so she has filed for divorce. He has two small children, ages 7 and 9 years.

Mental health experts from across the country predict that the psychiatric repercussions from Hurricane Katrina are likely to be far greater than anyone has ever seen [3,4]. With more than 1 million people displaced by Katrina, property destroyed or badly damaged, and more than 400,000 jobs lost, including those with health benefits, the predicted numbers of those who are or will be diagnosed with severe stress disorders is expected to be significant [3,4].

## Description

PTSD is distinguished from most mental health diagnoses in that it is tied to a particular traumatic life experience, which often involves intense fear of loss of life or serious injury. The disorder, which is also seen among rape victims and soldiers in combat, can occur any time after a trauma, with symptoms that include crippling panic attacks and terrifyingly vivid flashbacks that often last for years [5,6]. Studies have found that the longer individuals have been exposed to a threat of potential loss of life, the greater the likelihood they will develop PTSD [5,7,8]. The literature also shows that PTSD commonly occurs among people who are socially isolated, have

* Corresponding author.
E-mail address: jrhoad@lsuhsc.edu (J. Rhoads).

a history of psychological or physical trauma, and have preexisting mental health problems, such as depression or anxiety [6–9].

## Stress reactions

Many people most affected by Hurricane Katrina most likely experienced one or more of the four common stress reactions for several days and possibly weeks after the storm. The first common stress reaction is a psychological reaction that lasts several days or a couple of weeks and brings feelings of shock, fear, grief, anger, resentment, guilt, shame, helplessness, hopelessness, or emotional numbness (eg, difficulty in feeling love and intimacy or difficulty in taking an interest and experiencing pleasure with day-to-day activities) [9,10]. The second stress reaction is cognitive, and causes confusion, disorientation, and indecisiveness. Patients worry over small things and have a shortened attention span, difficulty concentrating, memory loss, or unwanted memories. In many cases, patients blame themselves for the bad things that happened [9,10].

Physical complaints are the third most common type of stress reaction. In these instances, patients complain of fatigue, edginess, difficulty sleeping, myalgia, pain, tachycardia, nausea, a change in appetite, or a change in sex drive. The last common stress reaction is psychosocial. This reaction is evident when patients avoid large crowds or socializing where they may be asked about the event. Work is often impaired; they may often call in sick to avoid any chances of exposure to anything that will remind them of the event [9,10]. Survivors have few friends because of poor interpersonal relationships at school, at work, or in their marriage. They distrust what others say and isolate themselves from anything that might remind them of the trauma they experienced [9,10]. Most people who experienced Hurricane Katrina will probably only have normal stress reactions. The literature documents that disaster experiences can often promote personal growth and strengthen relationships. However, one out of every three people who survived the disaster is likely to experience symptoms of PTSD [4,6].

## Epidemiology

Undoubtedly, the experiences of the people of New Orleans place them at a higher-than-normal risk for PTSD, especially those who had a history of exposure to disasters or traumas (eg, severe accidents, sexual or mental abuse, violence, combat, rescue work); chronic medical illness or psychological disorders; chronic poverty, homelessness, unemployment, or discrimination; or recent or subsequent major life stressors or emotional strain (eg, single parenting) [11]. Thus, these events involve actual or threatened death, injury, or threats to the integrity of self or others. In response to these events, the person experiences intense fear, helplessness, or horror. Memories of other times or traumas will resurface and only intensify current problems. Two other important aspects to consider when diagnosing PTSD is the age of the survivors when exposed to the trauma and level of education, which can make an individual more vulnerable to stress and reduce their ability to cope in highly stressful situations. Additional factors that increase risk for PTSD include "severity of initial reaction; peri-traumatic dissociation (ie, feeling numb and having a sense of unreality during and shortly following a trauma); early conduct problems; childhood adversity; family history of psychiatric disorder; poor social support after a trauma; and personality traits such as hypersensitivity, pessimism, and negative reactions to stressors" [10,11].

Several studies identified women as a high-risk group and found that they are more likely to develop PTSD than men, independent of any exposure to trauma or level of stress experienced [6–9]. Also, a previous history of depression increases women's vulnerability for developing PTSD [6–9].

Although traumatic events may increase vulnerability to subsequent traumas, research shows that exposure to trauma can have an inoculation effect and can even strengthen an individual's protective factors [6–9]. This reaction could occur because individuals have gained experience in mastering traumatic events successfully [6–9]. Survivor characteristics, such as gender and age, predisaster mental health and personality traits, and postdisaster psychosocial resources, also influence response to a traumatic event [10].

Cultural studies from Hurricane Andrew showed that Mexican more than Anglo-American women experienced PTSD, yet the incidence of PTSD in Anglo-American women was greater than in African-Americans [6–10]. School-aged children show greater psychological impairment after disasters such as these compared with adults [11–15]. Longitudinal studies of young children and adolescents exposed to Hurricane Andrew found that young individuals are at greater risk for postdisaster PTSD than older adults [11–15].

Several factors can aggravate stress reactions and increase the risk for developing negative outcomes, whereas others provide positive outcomes (Table 1) [12]. Examples of negative forces include poor coping strategies before the event, bad experiences at the scene of the disaster, lack of information about the disaster, and impersonal attention to the victims [12]. Positive forces also exist. A study of firefighters showed that psychosocial resources, such as hardiness, perceived control, and social support, afford critical protection for disaster victims [11].

## Screening

Paul is seen by a psychiatric mental health nurse practitioner who completes a physical examination and diagnostic workup that included a complete blood cell count with differential, complete metabolic screen, thyroid function studies, and drug screen. The examination results are all within normal limits. The mental status examination shows that Paul had feelings of guilt related to his choice not to be with his family, rejection by his peers because of his angry outbursts and rigidity, new onset of panic attacks whenever he embarks on a water search and rescue mission, intrusive thoughts of past rescues, and nightmares of all the dead bodies he retrieved from destroyed homes. Over the past 4 months he reports increased alcohol use and even tried smoking marijuana, hoping it would help him sleep. He denies the use of any other drug to aid his sleep.

Often people who have PTSD seek care for their complaints through their primary care provider (PCP) rather than from a psychologist or psychiatrist. They often complain of stomach ailments, insomnia, headaches, and pain. The PCP must be aware of the screening methods used to diagnose PTSD, because failure to do so could result in delayed diagnosis and treatment. Friedman [16], a psychiatrist and pharmacologist with the National Center for PTSD, developed a screening tool for PTSD, as shown in Box 1. It is a series of brief, problem-focused questions used in primary care and other medical settings. When patients give a positive answer to any three of the four questions, they must be screened

Table 1
Risk factors

| Increases risk | Decreases risk |
|---|---|
| • Little emotional and social support<br>• Presence of other stressors such as fatigue, cold, hunger, fear, uncertainty, loss, dislocation, and other psychologically stressful experiences<br>• Difficulties at the scene<br>• Lack of information about the nature and reasons for the event<br>• Lack of or interference with self-determination and self-management<br>• Treatment [given] in an authoritarian or impersonal manner<br>• Little follow-up support in the weeks after exposure<br>• Female gender<br>• Age of 40 to 60 years<br>• Ethnic minority<br>• Low socioeconomic status<br>• Children present in the home<br>• Presence of a husband who is significantly distressed<br>• Psychiatric history<br>• Severe exposure to the disaster, especially injury, life threat, and extreme loss<br>• Living in a highly disrupted or traumatized community<br>• Loss of money, home, car | • Social support<br>• Higher income and education<br>• Successful mastery of past disasters and traumatic events<br>• Limitation or reduction of exposure to any of the aggravating factors listed above<br>• Provision of information about expectations and availability of recovery services<br>• Care, concern, and understanding on the part of the recovery services personnel<br>• Provision of regular and appropriate information concerning the emergency and reasons for action |

*Data from* NSW Institute of Psychiatry and Centre for Mental Health. Disaster mental health response handbook. 2000; p. 33. NSW Health. North Sydney.

**Box 1. Friedman primary care posttraumatic stress disorder screen [17]**

In your life, have you ever had any experience that was so frightening, horrible, or upsetting that, *in the past month,* you...
1. Have had nightmares about it or thought about it when you did not want to? YES NO
2. Tried hard not to think about it or went out of your way to avoid situations that reminded you of it? YES NO
3. Were constantly on guard, watchful, or easily startled? YES NO
4. Felt numb or detached from others, activities, or your surroundings? YES NO

---

Current research suggests that the results of the PC-PTSD should be considered "positive" if a patient answers, "yes" to 3 out of 4 items.

*Data from* Foa E, Keane T, Friedman MJ. Treatments for PTSD: practice guidelines from the international society for traumatic stress studies, The Guilford Press. New York. 2000. p. 380.

symptoms along with severe distress, impairment, and dysfunction" [18]. Many mental health care providers use this tool as an aid in screening for PTSD [18,19].

**Diagnosis**

Paul is diagnosed with PTSD. His diagnosis is based on the following evidence: three re-experiencing symptoms (panic attacks, angry outbursts, and insomnia), three avoidance symptoms (avoiding water rescues, time with his family, and conversations related to past traumatic events), and two arousal symptoms (insomnia and angry outbursts), along with increasing use of alcohol, use of marijuana, and inability to sleep.

The term *PTSD* was first used in 1980, with four specific criteria [10,18].

*Criterion A: initial response to trauma*

The PCP must review the experiences regarding the traumatic event. The horror, helplessness, or fear patients may have experienced will provide an idea of the extent of the trauma.

*Criterion B: intrusive recollections*

With intrusive recollections, patients describe experiences as recurrent and have harsh flashbacks of the event. These flashbacks will be so intense that they may make them feel as if they are truly re-experiencing the traumatic event. Intense psychological distress will occur whenever patients are exposed to anything that resembles an aspect of the traumatic event. They describe feelings of rapid heart rates and the typical "fight or flight" phenomenon that often accompanies exposure to situations where life is endangered [10,18].

*Criterion C: numbing and withdrawal*

With criterion C, the provider diagnoses PTSD when patients begin to focus on anything to avoid any reminders of the trauma. Patients often state they feel numb or not attached to their bodies (dissociation). Responses are delayed, and patients block any thoughts, feelings, or conversations associated with the trauma [10,18]. They also avoid any activities, places, or people who might cause them to recollect the trauma, have no interest in participating in any social activities, and feel detached and isolated from others. Emotions are flat, and expressions of love or joy are

further for PTSD and should probably be referred to a mental health specialist; however, a positive response to the screen does not necessarily indicate that a patient has PTSD.

Dr. Edna Foa [17], a psychologist and professor at the University of Pennsylvania, also developed a PTSD questionnaire entitled *The Posttraumatic Stress Diagnostic Scale (PDS)* assessment, available through Pearson Assessments. The tool was designed to help detect and diagnose PTSD. The PDS assessment is aligned with diagnostic criteria from the *Diagnostic and Statistical Manual of Mental Disorders, Fourth Edition* (DSM-IV), and can be administered repeatedly over time to help screen for the presence of PTSD in large groups or in patients who have identified themselves as victims of a traumatic event. It is also a valuable tool to gauge symptom severity and functioning in patients already identified as experiencing PTSD [17,18].

For patients to be diagnosed with PTSD, they must have at "least one re-experiencing symptom, three avoidance symptoms, and two arousal nonexistent. They may feel hopeless and believe they face a depressing future (eg, do not expect to have a career, marriage, children, or normal lifespan) [10,18].

*Criterion D: persistent symptoms of increased arousal*

In this category, patients have repeated symptoms of heightened emotional states, such as anger or sadness. Subsequently, they experience difficulty falling or staying asleep, irritability or frequent outbursts of anger, difficulty concentrating, hypervigilance, or exaggerated startle responses [10,18].

The DSM-IV, Text Revision, diagnostic criteria for PTSD (309.81) stipulates that the patient must have been exposed to a traumatic event with at least one symptom from the re-experiencing or intrusion symptom cluster, three from numbing withdrawal symptom cluster, and one from the increased arousal symptom cluster. These symptoms must have been present for more than a month, resulting in clinically significant distress or impairment in social, occupational, or other important areas of functioning. Patients who fulfill these criteria are diagnosed with PTSD [10,18]. PTSD is considered acute if the symptoms last less than 3 months, or chronic if they persist longer than 3 months. Onset is occasionally considered delayed if symptoms appear at least 6 months after the stressor.

## Therapeutic interventions

Three weeks after Paul's diagnosis, he was placed on a selective serotonin reuptake inhibitor (SSRI) and assigned to a PTSD group therapy session. He also has attended weekly follow-up appointments with his provider to ensure he is tolerating the SSRI and benefiting from the group sessions. After 2 weeks, he reported progress in his recovery, evidenced by the fact that he was able to sleep through most of the night without intrusive thoughts, had no angry outbursts, and was able to understand his feelings about the storms' effect on him and his family. He arranged visits to his family and, with the help of family therapy, has been able to reconcile with his wife.

Therapeutic interventions used to treat PTSD are complex in terms of available treatments and their possible side effects. Once the PTSD diagnosis is made, the PCP should refer patients to a mental health care provider (MHCP) who will determine the severity of the PTSD according to the number of times they were exposed to the trauma, whether it is acute or chronic, and their gender and age. Once this information is verified, the most effective treatment that best fits the situation can be determined. Including the whole family unit provides the most effective treatment plan [17,18].

Therapies for PTSD may be divided into two distinctly different interventions: psychotherapies and pharmacotherapies [1,18]. Patients who have PTSD should be aware of all available therapeutic options and how effective each is for treating PTSD [17,18]. They should also know the general advantages and disadvantages (including side-effects) associated with each therapy.

*Psychotherapy*

Psychotherapeutic interventions have been used for many years and have proven effective, some more than others. Six therapies are discussed in this section.

*Cognitive therapy*

Cognitive therapy is a structured, short-term, present-oriented psychotherapy for depression [19,20]. This approach is used to help patients improve their moods through modifying dysfunctional thinking and behavior. Cognitive therapy for PTSD typically begins by helping patients understand how thoughts affect emotions and behavior. New skills are taught to help patients identify and clarify patterns of thinking. Studies show that cognitive therapy is an effective intervention for patients who have PTSD, primarily because it reduces survival guilt, self-blame, feelings of inadequacy, and worries about the future [20].

*Exposure therapy*

Exposure therapy helps reduce fear associated with experience through repetitive, therapist-guided confrontation of the places or things that constitute the traumatic event [19–21]. Exposure therapy usually lasts from 8 to 12 sessions, depending on how severe the PTSD is, and incorporates factors such as age and physical and mental health of the individual. Patients are repeatedly exposed to the fear stimuli until their symptoms (eg, arousal, fear responses) decrease [19–21]. Female victims of sexual and mental abuse, motor vehicle accident victims, men and women in military combat, and trauma cases have all been shown to benefit from exposure therapy, [19–21].

However, cases exist where exposure therapy is contraindicated. All patients must be carefully screened to determine whether the level of distress that normally results from exposure therapy would be detrimental. Patients who reside in threatening environments are not candidates for exposure therapy until their security can be assured, because this treatment may increase distress and heighten PTSD symptoms [19–21]. Also, patients may feel uncomfortable with exposure therapy and discontinue treatment [19–21]. Practitioners must carefully educate all patients about any treatment, providing clear rationale for the treatment, exploring any patient concerns, encouraging realistic goals, and subsequently building a strong commitment to the therapy. All this will reduce the risk for dropout [19–21].

*Stress inoculation training*

Stress inoculation training (SIT) was developed to manage anxiety symptoms. It was originally designed to treat female rape trauma survivors [19,20]. SIT typically consists of "education and training of coping skills, including deep muscle relaxation training, breathing control, assertiveness, role playing, covert modeling, thought stopping, positive thinking and self-talk" [19,20]. The premise in this treatment is that trauma-related anxiety can be generalized to many situations [19–21]. This therapy builds on well-validated cognitive–behavioral techniques. Its goal is to "inoculate" individuals to situations that can reactivate their trauma, causing symptoms of anxiety, depression, and distress.

*Eye movement desensitization and reprocessing*

Eye movement desensitization and reprocessing (EMDR) is a treatment used to assist patients in alleviating the distress connected with traumatic memories [22]. Dr. Francine Shapiro [22] developed the treatment to help patients examine and process traumatic memories so that they do not evoke stressful recollections or other debilitating symptoms [22]. Evidence shows significant clinical improvements with PTSD symptoms after only a few sessions with EMDR. Overall, EMDR research has been shown to have variable findings associated with its efficacy [22].

*Imagery rehearsal therapy*

Most patients with PTSD complain of nightmares and disturbing dreams. The literature shows that 4% to 8% of the general population,

but as many as 60% of those who have PTSD, experience these sleep disturbances.

Imagery rehearsal therapy (IRT) focuses on changing the images in nightmares to those that are rewarding rather than threatening. The patient then has mastery and control over the event. The small amount of clinical trial research reports significant reductions in nightmares and improvements in PTSD and comorbid symptomatology [19,20].

*Psychodynamic psychotherapy*

Psychodynamic psychotherapy is "an interaction between a psychotherapist and a client that leads to changes—from a less adaptive state to a more adaptive state—in the client's thoughts, feelings, and behaviors" [20]. The theory behind this therapy stresses the importance of addressing unconscious mental feelings and emotions so the patient can learn how to cope with the effects of PTSD [20]. With this therapy, the therapist explores fears, fantasies, and defenses inspired by the traumatic event and incorporates supportive and expressive translation of these findings. Psychodynamic psychotherapy has been documented to be more effective than the other treatments, because it significantly improves coping skills and increases self-esteem [20].

*Group therapy*

The main objective of group therapy is to provide a supportive environment in which patients who have PTSD can receive help together. Group therapy first began in the 1970s and was used to help patients address their symptoms of "isolation, alienation, and diminished feelings" [19,20]. Group therapy creates an environment in which patients help each other. Group approaches are characterized as "supportive," "psychodynamic," or "cognitive–behavioral" [19].

*Pharmacotherapeutics*

Most health care providers are very aware that any kind of stress reaction can cause biologic, psychological, and behavioral changes. The biologic changes can disrupt sleep patterns or produce heightened physical and emotional responses, such as pain and gastrointestinal symptoms [18–20]. Psychologically, patients complain of mood disturbances (eg, labiality, irritability, blunting, numbing), anxiety (eg, increased worry, ruminations), and cognitive disturbances (eg, memory impairment, confusion, impaired task completion) [17–19]. If treatment fails to improve symptoms and all possible medical diagnoses have been ruled out, medications may be considered [17–19]. If medications are indicated, the goal should be to select the optimal agent with as few adverse effects as possible.

Antidepressants, tricyclic antidepressants (TCAs), monoamine oxidase inhibitors (MAOIs), selective serotonin reuptake inhibitors (SSRIs), antianxiety and adrenergic agents, and mood stabilizers have all been used to treat PTSD [17–19]. The SSRIs, specifically paroxetine and sertraline, are shown to be the most effective in treating PTSD [17–19]. Both drugs have produced clinical improvements in several randomized clinical trials among patients who have PTSD [17–19]. Olanzapine, which was used with significant results to treat afflicted Korean veterans [17–19], is another SSRI used to treat PTSD. Olanzapine and fluphenazine have also been used successfully to treat combat-induced PTSD in individuals from the Balkans. Both medicines successfully improved PTSD and psychotic symptomatology [17–19].

## Patient education

With patient education, therapists provide a therapeutic environment so that communication is freely exchanged and the symptoms and functional impairments of PTSD are reduced. *Psychoeducation* is a broad term that is often included as a component of other psychiatric education used to assist families in understanding PTSD and exploring the various treatments available [20,21]. In addition to education, therapists provide support to patients, informing them that the conditions can and will improve with time and treatment [20]. Education about the symptoms and treatment of comorbid disorders may also be included [20]. Families are an extremely important part of the education process, and therefore all PTSD treatment and intervention efforts must educate the entire family and significant others. Outreach efforts for intensive services should focus on locations where at-risk individuals and families are most likely to live [20], and treatments and interventions known to be effective should be implemented. Encouragement must be provided to families, especially spouses and mothers, because managing children who have PTSD requires special skills.

## Care of children who have posttraumatic stress disorder

Children and adolescents who have experienced a trauma such as hurricane Katrina must be evaluated carefully, because the way they display symptoms of distress may change as they age. Additionally, severity and proximity of and parental reaction to the traumatic event may place the child at greater risk for PTSD [14,15]. Younger children may act out their symptoms through play or drawing. They may experience a feeling of a foreshortened future and missequenced events (known as "time skew") and identify forerunners of the traumatic event (known as "omen formation"). Regressive behaviors, such as thumb sucking and enuresis, may be apparent [14,15]. Increased impulsivity and a tendency to isolate may be noted, especially among adolescents [15] because they are more inclined to display aggressive behaviors and may reenact some aspects of the trauma in their daily lives [13]. Children and adolescents who have experienced major traumas such as Hurricane Katrina may exhibit symptoms of other psychiatric disorders, such as generalized anxiety, depression, substance abuse, oppositional defiant disorder, and conduct disorder [13]. The event may be discussed gradually with relaxation techniques and anxiety management.

Treatment of PTSD in children and adolescents may include individual, group, and family therapy. For children and adolescents who have PTSD, pharmacotherapy focuses on the treatment of specific symptoms and is somewhat limited [15]. Despite of the shortage of randomized controlled trials, SSRIs may be considered a good first choice for treating the core symptoms of PTSD, such as anxiety, mood, and re-experiencing of symptoms, whereas adrenergic agents such as clonidine may be used for problems with impulsivity and hyperarousal. Any decision to put children on SSRIs should be approached cautiously and after consulting with a psychiatrist (or other credentialed provider) and the family about the associated risks and benefits. Atypical neuroleptics may help manage severe self-injurious activities and dissociation, aggression, and psychosis [23]. Cognitive–behavioral therapy has been used effectively for some children and adolescents [21]. Play therapy is useful for younger children who may be unable to verbalize their feelings. Psychoeducation on the symptoms and effects of PTSD is helpful for parents, because it enables them to better understand the trauma and its effects and makes them more able to support the child and improve functioning [15]. EMDR has been used in children with some success [15].

## Summary

Paul's last visit to the clinic was a happy one. His wife and family came to New Orleans to meet with the nurse practitioner and they participated in family counseling sessions. As a result, Paul and his wife have reconciled and he will be moving to Houston to be with them. His nurse practitioner scheduled a follow-up appointment for Paul at a mental health care clinic in Houston and confirms all of Paul's records will be sent to his new provider.

People cannot completely protect themselves from traumatic experiences. Up to 8% [6] of individuals will experience PTSD in their lives, and everyone would most likely develop PTSD if exposed to severe-enough trauma. It is most important to quickly recognize the signs and symptoms of PTSD. Prompt recognition will enable providers to act quickly with the appropriate treatment modalities, improve quality of life, and prevent disability and recurrence, all of which will at least disrupt and may even end a person's life if unrecognized and untreated.

## References

[1] Katrina. USA Today. September 2005. Available at: www.usatoday.com Accessed October, 2005.

[2] Koopman C, Classen CC, Cardena E, et al. When disaster strikes, acute stress disorder may follow. J Trauma Stress 1995;8(1):29–46.

[3] Cappiello J. Assessing public health and the delivery of care in the wake of Katrina. Washington, DC: Joint Commission on Accreditation of Healthcare Organizations; September 22, 2005 Available at: http://energycommerce.house.gov/108/Hearings/09222005hearing1643/Cappiello2617.htm Accessed July 19, 2006.

[4] Watanabe M. Post Katrina medicine: be aware of symptoms of traumatic stress. Applied Neurology 2005; Available at: http://www.aaneurology.com/article/printableArticle.jhtml?articleId=175400212&. Accessed November 16, 2006 printable.

[5] Norris FH, Friedman MJ, Watson PJ. 60,000 disaster victims speak: part II, summary and implications of the disaster mental health research. Psychiatry 2005;65(3):240–60.

[6] National Center for PTSD. Facts about PTSD. 2005. Available at: http://www.ncptsd.va.gov/. Accessed December 19, 2006.

[7] Bryant RA, Harvey AG. Acute stress disorder: a critical review of diagnostic issues. Clin Psychol Rev 1997;17:757–73.

[8] Kessler RC, Sonnega A, Bromet EJ, et al. Posttraumatic stress disorder in the national comorbidity survey. Arch Gen Psychiatry 1995;52(12):1048–60.

[9] Brady KT. Posttraumatic stress disorder and comorbidity: recognizing the many faces of PTSD. J Clin Psychiatry 1997;58(Suppl 9):12–5.

[10] Blank AS Jr. Clinical detection, diagnosis, and differential diagnosis of post-traumatic stress disorder. Psychiatr Clin North Am 1994;17:351–83.

[11] van der Kolk AC, Bessel A. History of trauma in psychiatry. In: van der Kolk Bessel A, McFarlane Alexander C, Weisaeth Lars, editors. Traumatic stress: the effects of overwhelming experience on mind, body, and society. New York: The Guilford Press; 1996. p. 367–78.

[12] NSW Institute of Psychiatry and Centre for Mental Health. Disaster mental health response handbook. North Sydney: NSW Health; 2000.

[13] Lubit R. PTSD in children. Emedicine May 3, 2006; Available at: http://www.emedicine.com/ped/topic3026.htm Accessed November 16, 2006.

[14] Anderson T. PTSD in children and adolescents. Chicago: University of Illinois; 2005 (Great Cities Institute MC107)College of Urban Planning and Public Affairs. Great Cities Institute Publication Number: GCP-05-04.

[15] Hamblen J. PTSD in Children and adolescents. United States Department of Veteran Affairs. National Center for PTSD; 2006 Available at: http://ncptsd.va.gov/facts/specific/fs_children.html. Accessed November 16, 2006.

[16] Friedman MJ. Current and future drug treatment for posttraumatic stress disorder patients. Psychiatr Ann 1998;28:461–8.

[17] Foa E, Keane T, Friedman MJ. Treatments for PTSD: practice guidelines from the international society for traumatic stress studies. New York: The Guilford Press; 2000.

[18] Foa E, Cahill SP, Boscarino JA. Social, psychological, and psychiatric interventions following terrorist attacks: recommendations for practice and research. Neuropsychopharmacology 2005;30:1806–17.

[19] Richmond RL. Types of psychological treatment. A guide to psychology and its practice 19 March 2006; Available at: www.guidetopsychology.com Accessed November 16, 2006.

[20] Lovell K, Marks IM, Noshirvani H, et al. Do cognitive and exposure treatments improve various PTSD symptoms differently? A randomized controlled trial. Behavioral and Cognitive Psychotherapy 2001;29(1):107–12.

[21] Shapiro F. Eye movement desensitization and reprocessing: basic principles, protocols and procedures. 2nd edition. New York: Guilford Press; 2001.

[22] Donnelly CL. Pharmacologic treatment approaches for children and adolescents with posttraumatic stress disorder. Child Adolesc Psychiatr Clin N Am 2003;12(2):251–64.

[23] Ursano RJ, Grieger TA, McCarroll JE. Prevention of posttraumatic stress: consultation, training, and early treatment. In: Van der Kolk BA, McFarlane AC, Weisaeth L, editors. Traumatic stress: the effects of overwhelming experience on mind, body, and society. New York: Guilford Press; 1996. p. 441–62.

ELSEVIER
SAUNDERS

Crit Care Nurs Clin N Am 20 (2008) 83–90

CRITICAL CARE
NURSING CLINICS
OF NORTH AMERICA

# Caring for the Caregivers and Patients Left Behind: Experiences of a Volunteer Nurse During Hurricane Katrina

## Sandra L. Leiby, RN, MSN, APRN-BC

*Graduate School of Nursing, University of Massachusetts, 55 Lake Avenue North,*
*Worcester, MA 01655, USA*

Hurricane Katrina, a category five storm, hit the Gulf Coast region of the United States on August 29, 2005, and ravaged more than 90,000 square miles, destroyed billions of dollars of property, and crippled a major American city. This natural disaster was the most devastating and costliest in American history [1]. The region was left with thousands of homeless families; thousands of persons were killed, and hundreds of thousands were evacuated [2]. Medical facilities were crippled by a lack of electric power, potable water, and essential services. New Orleans medical facilities and hospitals were on the front lines of the crisis.

During the days and weeks after Hurricane Katrina, the media coverage showed families sitting on the roofs of their flooded homes, countless thousands stranded at the Superdome and Convention Center without food and drinkable water, and masses evacuated with no homes to which to return. While watching the newscasts, I thought that the people of New Orleans and the surrounding region were going to be in great need of medical and nursing care. Reports of damaged and destroyed medical facilities and the mass evacuation of patients and staff fueled my desire to offer my nursing skills to that devastated area. During the continual news updates, volunteer organization Websites and phone numbers were offered for a wide variety of services. I volunteered on-line for the American Red Cross [3] and the Hurricane Katrina Health Care Professionals

and Relief Workers with the US Department of Health and Human Services (DHHS) [4]. This step marked the beginning of a journey on which I ultimately learned many lessons, including the necessity for clear communication and leadership, volunteer flexibility with an "I'll-do-anything" mind-set, and more disaster training to ensure organizational and personal preparedness. This article describes my experiences and highlights how I learned those lessons as a volunteer nurse after Hurricane Katrina.

## The volunteer process

Having a background in volunteering and international nursing with underserved populations, I thought that I possessed the skills needed for this type of relief work. I filled out on-line applications to have my Massachusetts nursing license credentialed. Periodically, I provided updates on needed information. As the media coverage on the devastation and magnitude of human suffering unfolded, I felt in a small way that I was being productive. In the meantime, I donated bags of clothes, shampoo, and cases of baby food to a local drive for Katrina victims.

The first response to my volunteer application arrived about 3 weeks later. On September 24, 2005, I received an e-mail from a Public Health Service Commander, Office of the US Surgeon General, Public Health Service (PHS), alerting me that I was to be a part of a deployment team for Katrina Relief. More details concerning my deployment would arrive within 48 hours. One week later, when I still had not heard any more news on

*E-mail address:* sandra.leiby@umassmed.edu

0899-5885/08/$ - see front matter © 2008 Elsevier Inc. All rights reserved.
doi:10.1016/j.ccell.2007.10.007

*ccnursing.theclinics.com*

a deployment, I disappointedly put the issue to the back of my mind, and continued with my busy life. Seven days later, the call to deploy arrived. It was Saturday, October 1 at 10 PM. The Commander asked if I could be ready for deployment on October 3, at 6 AM. With only 68 hours' notice, being enrolled full time in graduate school courses, working as a staff registered nurse, and teaching in an associate-degree nursing program, I did not feel that I could leave all my responsibilities that suddenly. Thus, I declined to deploy and e-mailed my professors, nurse manager, and students about my decision. My inbox immediately filled with e-mails unanimously encouraging me to accept the chance to deploy. To do their part in helping those affected by Hurricane Katrina, my professors and clinical preceptors remained flexible with make-up work, colleagues covered all my work shifts, and my students helped to rearrange my teaching schedule. With this show of support, I called the Commander to accept the deployment.

According to the DHHS Website [5], more than "33,000 health care professional and relief personnel had registered with the [DHHS] for possible deployment in affected areas." Later, I found out that I was one of only 1000 medical professionals chosen for this mission. Fortunately, my deployment team was delayed for 2 days, so I had enough time to gather up my needed equipment for the trip, including boots, gloves, masks, insect spray, and nursing supplies. Through telephone calls, e-mails and the DHHS Website, I learned that I needed to "be healthy enough to function under field conditions" and "that the work may include 12-hour shifts, austere conditions (eg, possibility of no showers and living in tents), no air conditioning, long periods of standing, sleeping accommodations on a bed roll, military ready-to-eat-meals, and portable toilets" [5].

### Deployment to Louisiana

Armed with two suitcases full of nursing supplies and personal items, I was off to Lafayette, Louisiana: mission unknown. After arriving at the Lafayette airport, I boarded a bus with four other nurses. For the next 4 hours, we traveled from the airport to a military base to pick up another 20 nurses, physicians, pharmacists, and physical therapists. Eventually, we ended up at Camp Allen in Baton Rouge, Louisiana, where I remained for 48 hours. During that time, I was "federalized" (meaning I was placed under the

federal government's control, allowing me, through the Federal Emergency Management Agency [FEMA], to practice as a registered nurse in Louisiana with an out-of-state license). I then waited to find out my role.

Camp Allen was equipped with 15 large circus tents that each could accommodate 100 military cots. My co-ed tent housed nurses, physicians, DHHS employees, civilians, and other allied health personnel from all over the country. After my first night sleeping on a military cot, showering in a trailer bed converted into a shower facility, and using one of the 102 portable toilets lined up in our camp, I gathered in a tent with the rest of the volunteers and our commanding staff from DHHS.

During our first meeting with staff officials from DHHS, our commanders announced the needs in the area and asked us to organize into small groups based on medical or nursing specialty. We used loose-leaf binder paper to make signs to label our specialties: critical care, telemetry, medical/surgical, pharmacy, and mortuary, among others. Based on these specialties, we divided ourselves into sections, only to be told that we needed to organize by different groups. We repeated this process during that meeting and the many similar meetings that followed.

At these meetings I began to learn many lessons about the need for communication, organization, and planning. My prior military experience had made me familiar with the phrase, "hurry up and wait": one rushes to a meeting only to stand around and wait for a long time, while officials sort out deployment plans. Most of the other volunteers did not have this experience, however, and they expected to be moved out into the community immediately, helping and meeting the needs of the people we had seen in the media for so many weeks. They had little patience with the conflicting announcements and grew drained and weary. Some became angry.

The confusion about deployment priorities clearly arose from lack of coordination between local and state officials and with our DHHS staff. Despite the great needs of the communities in the Gulf Coast region, the mission and goals of disaster relief were neither clearly defined nor readily communicated to the volunteers. The relief workers and government representatives were genuinely concerned and unselfishly desired to help in this huge humanitarian crisis, but a system for disaster relief that could meet the community's needs quickly was not in place. This experience raised my awareness of the importance of advanced preparation and planning for contingencies, clear communication, and effective leadership.

Another area that the deployment process failed to address was educating the volunteers regarding the command structure that would be managing the aftermath of the flood and organizing the relief work, and explaining how the volunteers fit into that structure. Thus, it was unclear to the volunteers how FEMA, DHHS, PHS, and all the other organizations "with initials" were coordinating their efforts and what specific roles each played. During meetings, countless uniformed officials would brief us on another possible plan for the volunteers. This lack of coordination and clear direction made the volunteers wonder aloud, "Who is in charge?", "What is our mission?", and "Which organization is which?" [6]. We now know that many of these concerns and issues have been the focus of many high-level government discussions during the sessions considering the lessons learned from Hurricanes Katrina and Rita [7].

## Our mission: staffing one of few functioning hospitals in New Orleans

Finally, on day three of my deployment, I was assigned with 19 other nurses to a group called "ARF 154" (a designation that was never explained). Our mission was to work as telemetry nurses at a hospital in the suburbs of New Orleans. We designated one nurse as our leader, with responsibility for coordinating communication between the PHS staff and our group. During our 90-minute trip south, we introduced ourselves and found that we hailed geographically from Hawaii to Boston, with levels of expertise ranging from new graduate to semi-retired nurses and nurse practitioners with more than 30 years of experience.

This destination hospital, located on the west bank of the Mississippi River, was one of few hospitals among the area's 13 medical facilities that were still open 6 weeks after Katrina. As we disembarked from our vans, the Disaster Medical Assistance Team (DMAT) from Toledo, Ohio greeted us. The team, which was set up in the hospital's parking lot and watched over by the National Guard, was responsible for triaging patients before they entered the hospital emergency room. When I entered the hospital—a clean, undamaged, beautiful medical facility—I was confused and questioned the need for our deployment. After meeting hospital officials, presenting our nursing credentials and identification,

eating dinner in the hospital cafeteria, and receiving our nursing assignments, we loaded our belongings onto a bus and were transferred to our new housing facility.

On a 10-minute drive down the highway and past a few side streets, we saw mostly deserted streets, closed businesses, uprooted trees, boarded windows, and blue tarps on most roofs. We arrived at our destination, a nonfunctioning hospital, only a few miles from downtown New Orleans. This hospital, which became the new home we would share with the National Guard, Veterans Administration Nurses, and displaced hospital workers, had been taken over by the parish government and served as headquarters for the National Guard. It was surreal to take up residence on an inpatient hospital floor, two nurses per room, where we slept in hospital beds and were guarded by personnel in fatigues carrying rifles.

## My role as a volunteer nurse

My role within the hospital was similar to that at my home medical center. I shadowed a staff nurse for 1 day, watching direct patient care, medication distribution, and other floor-nursing skills for which I would be responsible. The next day I began working four consecutive 12-hour shifts, 1 day off, followed by an additional four consecutive 12-hour shifts. Once on the telemetry floor, I was relieved to discover many familiar tools and systems. The system used on the floor was similar to the medication-dispensing system with which I was familiar. In addition, the intravenous pumps, glucose-monitoring machine, and many patient supplies were identical to those I was accustomed to using. Patient records, notes, and flow sheet assessments used a paper system that was easy to navigate. The computer system, including the electronic medication administration record, was not user-friendly, however. Despite our lack of training in using the computer system, the volunteer nurses were expected to perform order entry and coordinate with dietary, transportation, and pharmacy. Clearly, documentation and procedures need to be standardized during disasters to help volunteers with the transition [8]. Nonetheless, these adjustments to system differences did not affect one-on-one patient care, which was the one constant and the focus of our efforts.

While working on the telemetry floor, I made many interesting observations of the staff nurses.

This institution's nursing staff had come from many area hospitals that had been destroyed or damaged in the storm. Most had experienced personal and property losses, or at least damage. All of them functioned with an uncertain financial or occupational future, and the work atmosphere was charged with an understandable underlying tension. This experience taught me the need for an "I'll-do-anything" mind-set. We volunteer nurses did routine work, much as on our own units at home. The hospital floors often were short-staffed, and we received little assistance with patient care. The volunteer nurses were not widely accepted by the floor nurses, because they assumed that FEMA was paying us handsomely for our work. I emphasized that I was receiving no compensation beyond my travel expenses, food, and a place to stay. I also pointed out that I was separated from my family, would receive no pay for my 2-week deployment, because I am a per-diem employee, and would have to make up all missing graduate school assignments and clinical teaching days. Once the staff understood the sacrifices made by the ARF 154 nurses, we were accepted more readily.

Nonetheless, many volunteer nurses in our group became disillusioned with our mission. Lacking contact with PHS and without any hospital liaison, we had no means for dealing with conflict or problems. Some volunteer nurses never felt accepted by the staff, and others thought that they were put in unsafe clinical situations. The simple issue of where to wash our scrubs became a problem with no real solution. Many volunteer nurses had thought our mission would involve roaming New Orleans streets to help the sick and hurt, work that was not needed 6 weeks after the storm. Traveling hundreds or thousands of miles to perform nursing duties that "could be done at home" disappointed some. This "disconnect between the aspirations of the army of volunteers and the actual needs of the victims of Hurricane Katrina" [9] was evident to all. This experience taught me that the role of a disaster volunteer is to fill whatever need presents itself, even though it might not coincide with preconceptions about that role.

**Patient stories**

Many of the patients shared their experiences with me. One of my patients was a 75-year-old woman who had diabetes. During our discussions, we realized that her house was directly behind the hospital where our volunteer group was living. The day before, I had been amazed by her house, a two-story home that was missing its roof and entire second floor. I had taken a picture of the house because it was so representative of the condition of the entire community. This woman had decided to weather the storm in her home, but when the upper floor was ripped from the house, she fled for safety to my living quarters. Six weeks after the storm, the woman was admitted with dangerously high blood glucose levels and blood pressure to the hospital where I was working. She had run out of insulin and antihypertensive medications, and with the health care system in upheaval, she was unable to reach her health care provider. I saw this patient on her second day after admission. Even though 6 weeks had passed since the storm, the night before had been the first time she had slept through the night since the hurricane. Because of hurricane-related events, this patient showed possible signs of posttraumatic stress syndrome and the ramifications of her disrupted health care regimen [10,11].

One 82-year-old man, who had been admitted with renal problems, reported staying behind during the storm to protect his property. Because of the looting after the flooding, this elderly man, who many comorbid medical issues, spent the night on the roof of his house armed with a rifle. He stated that he had to use this weapon "to show that he meant business." Another patient was a 77-year-old woman who had been admitted 2 weeks before my arrival. She had been triaged in the hospital parking lot by a DMAT team from Boston. Her medical condition had been life threatening, and she needed immediate surgery; she believed that the rapid care by the DMAT team saved her life. When she found out that I was a volunteer from Massachusetts, she kissed my face and hands as she thanked me with tears. I cried with her.

**Nursing staff stories**

My mind-set of "I'll do anything" led me to care not only for the patients left after the storm but also for the caregivers. The local nursing staffs were dealing with incredible adjustments and loss, including lost family members and homes. Some of the staff had been relocated from other facilities where they had built long-term working relationships. Many of their spouses had lost jobs, making these nurses the only family source of income and medical benefits [12]. Many days I overheard nurses on the phone with either the Red Cross or FEMA agencies, trying to rebuild their lives along with their homes. Some staff had to leave periodically to bury dead family members.

In the midst of my workday, I often asked the staff what had happened to them because of Katrina. On the surface, they seemed relaxed and focused on daily patient care. As the staff members shared their experiences and lives, I learned of the immense devastation each person was enduring. I saw that I was in a unique position. All the nursing staff shared the devastating experiences with which they were all living. I, on the other hand, offered a safe place to share their thoughts and feelings [11]. Every day, the staff and patients shared stories of tragedy and loss. At times, I would feel so overwhelmed with their accounts that I went on long walks for hours at a time [13]. I wanted to say, "No more!!!" I kept listening because I had made a commitment to meet whatever needs had to be filled.

The stories told of preparing for the storm, living through it, and dealing with its aftermath. Before the storm hit, the hospital discharged any patients that could be released. The National Guard was brought into the hospital before the storm to ensure security. Two family members were allowed to stay with the remaining patients through the hurricane; the National Guard escorted any additional family members out of the building. Many staff members signed up for "hurricane duty," because it included extra pay.

One licensed practical nurse led me by the hand into the room in the hospital where she had stayed during the worst of the storm. She described the storm sounding like a locomotive and the huge protective windows bowing, but never shattering. This nurse and those at other facilities recounted having no working toilet facilities and having to void and defecate into plastic bags, which then were collected in biohazard bags [14]. Food and water were rationed for patients and staff. The emergency generators could not handle the air-conditioning system, and temperatures within the facility rose to 110°F. Nurses cut their scrubs into shorts and sometimes had to be hooked up to intravenous fluids to perform patient care. Survival during the crisis was based not on institutional or medical management but on professionalism, personal preparedness, and professional and personal ethics [14].

While a young nurse and I were eating lunch, she began to tell me her story. She had stayed behind to do hurricane duty and found the experience unsettling. Toward the end of her story, she leaned forward and spoke very softly about rumors of euthanasia at another New Orleans Hospital. She talked about the difficulties of caring for critically ill patients with very limited resources at this institution. She shared the incredible burden she felt to provide competent nursing care, including effective life-sustaining measurements and pain management and said she could only imagine the ethical dilemma faced by the other hospital's staff [15]. I saw how some of the storm's effects and the choices that had to be made during the storm had wreaked a huge emotional toll on the medical staff. I could picture the dilemmas facing these health care professionals as I watched this nurse begin to cry, so overcome with emotion that she could no longer speak.

Another nurse recounted handing a baby, which had been under her care in the neonatal intensive care unit, to helicopter staff to be evacuated. She still had nagging questions surrounding the survival of that baby. We heard stories of physicians breaking into local pharmacies to find badly needed medical supplies [16]. Several nurses reported hearing gunshots outside the hospital and were thankful that the National Guard was within the facility to protect them; other hospitals were not as fortunate [10]. The staff nurses also were in the unique position of helping patients and their family members deal with loss and death, as they themselves were dealing with chaotic bereavement related to trauma and possible death of patients and their own family members [12].

Because most of the hospitals in New Orleans had been shut down and their staff transferred to our institution, some staff issues evolved. The "transplants" were dealing with leaving their workplaces and transitioning to new positions with new coworkers in a new work environment. Additionally, each staff member was experiencing various levels of storm-related stress, loss, and trauma.

## Downtown New Orleans

After working 4 days as a floor nurse, I accompanied several volunteer nurses into downtown New Orleans to see the devastation. We immediately realized that the people on the streets were predominantly relief workers, the National Guard, government officials, and the media. Our first stop was the Superdome. We walked around the stadium and saw the dark brown line on the walls leading up to the building, which showed how high the floodwaters had reached. The roof was still heavily damaged, and we could see mold and mildew through all the windows. The smell of rotting sewage permeated the air. By the time we had walked half way around the stadium, two men in HAZMAT gear emerged from the building. They quickly asked us to leave, telling us that we were walking on dried fecal matter and that the area had tested positive for tuberculosis [17].

We continued walking though the downtown area, passing the devastated Veteran's Hospital, Charity Hospital (the largest state-funded health sciences/level I trauma center) [18], Charity School of Nursing, and the Tulane University Hospital. The streets outside these facilities were strewn with abandoned boats, jet skis, and smashed automobiles. The receding floodwaters had left a watermark about waist high on all the buildings, and all vegetation below the flood level had died. The National Guard was patrolling the streets and passing out water and fruit to relief workers. Military aircraft continually flew overhead.

## St. Bernard's Parish

A few days before we were sent back to Baton Rouge and Camp Allen, 11 nurses from ARF 154 were allowed into St. Bernard's Parish. Touring the parish, we saw homes that had been under up to 10 feet of toxic floodwater for several weeks after the levees broke. Homes had been lifted from their foundations and floated blocks down the street, trucks were in swimming pools, cars were on cars, and cars were on houses. I took hundreds of photographs, none of which could capture the devastation accurately.

A pivotal moment for me was helping two families who had just been allowed to return to their homes 6 weeks after Katrina. Both homes had been flooded to the second floor, and the receding water had left approximately 8 inches of sludge that was reported to be full of toxic chemicals and human waste [19]. We nurses divided into two teams and began digging with shovels and wheelbarrows. Wearing scrubs, masks, gloves, and boots, we emptied the first floor of each home. The National Guard drove by periodically to provide water and military ready-to-eat meals. Every personal belonging in

the home was destroyed and was placed in a heap on the front lawn. While we shoveled the mud in the kitchen area of one home, rats ran through our feet. As I emptied books, clothes, plates, pots, and pans onto the front lawn, I gained an appreciation for the magnitude of loss experienced by the people of New Orleans.

## Need for disaster training

My time as a volunteer nurse after Hurricane Katrina taught me valuable personal and professional lessons. The greatest lesson was the need for training to ensure organizational and personal preparedness for future mass casualties or disasters. The issues that caused delays and miscommunication in deploying needed health care relief workers need to be understood to ensure that planners can consider those issues and avert negative outcomes in the future.

My deployment experiences clearly highlighted the lack of collaboration and clear communication between federal, state, and nongovernmental agencies during the hurricane aftermath. Media coverage of the devastation in the New Orleans area resulted in many clinicians self-deploying to the region, which only compounded the overall disorganization [9]. I could see the need for national standards on disaster or emergency management, operations, communication, accrediting personnel, resource and information management, and technology support.

Training of health care workers should include the Incident Command System (ICS) that outlines the command structure during a mass casualty event. This command system was created on February 28, 2003, by President Bush as part of the National Incident Management System (NIMS) to "provide a consistent nationwide template to enable all government, private-sector, and nongovernmental organizations to work together during domestic incidents" [20]. As of 2005, federal agencies require that state and local departments and agencies adopt the NIMS command structure to receive federal preparedness funding. Membership in many regional Medical Reserve Corps requires completing the on-line learning module IS700 NIMS, which outlines the ICS [21], Multi-agency Coordination Systems, and Public Information Systems. The recently finalized Hospital Emergency Incident Command System (HICS) [21] provides guidance for institutional disaster and emergency plans but needs to address standardization of communication and the use of clear language, because responders to future events will come from different states and possibly several nations [8,22]. The HICS also should include a standardized system for triaging disaster patients [15].

According to the Agency for Healthcare Research and Quality [23], health care providers cannot be assumed to know how to deliver appropriate care during disaster or mass casualty events. They must receive disaster training that includes culturally sensitive care of survivors and patients [13]. Training in ethical, moral, legal, medical, and group decision making can help responders during catastrophic events, when even the most seasoned professional may be rattled [15]. Because disasters require responders to practice in "unfamiliar and unusual conditions," the responders may need to adapt to more widely recognized standards of care [24]. Volunteers also need to be on a reasonable rotation schedule to prevent exhaustion and to avoid becoming casualties themselves [6]. Nurses can play a vital role in disaster preparedness [1], but they need to be trained specifically for disaster relief. To meet these training needs and to deal with the complexities of disaster-relief health care in the twenty-first century, government and nursing organizations need to develop high-quality, focused training and education programs [25]. "Disaster workers must be assured that they have the best information available about the potential hazards they may face, receive and use effective protective equipment, have appropriate health care and health monitoring, and be supported legally and ethically when making difficult clinical decisions. If we do not address these issues now, who will respond the next time?" [26].

Last, disaster preparedness must not overlook disaster volunteers' and responders' vital need for postdeployment support [25]. For several weeks after I returned from New Orleans, I was plagued by nightmares and problems sleeping as I continually relived my experiences [27,28]. Posttraumatic stress syndrome is more prevalent in the aftermath of a natural disaster than after any other type of trauma [10,29], but I did not have any debriefing or postdeployment follow-up. Although the value of compulsory debriefing for anyone exposed to a critical event is controversial [30–32], group debriefing of the ARF 154 nurses would have allowed us to understand some of the emotions and feelings we might experience in the aftermath of our deployment.

## Summary

In looking back at my experiences as a volunteer nurse deployed to New Orleans after Hurricane Katrina, I value every experience and lesson I learned. I feel honored to have been welcomed into so many lives at a point of intense suffering. Although the accounts of the experiences were often overwhelming, these stories are now a part of who I am. Some of the lessons I learned resulted from observing the man-made disaster that followed the natural disaster. These lessons included the need for honest and informative leadership [33], for volunteer flexibility and an "I'll-do-anything" mind-set, and for more advanced disaster training. Learning from the experiences of responders to recent national and international relief efforts will ensure organizational and personal preparedness needed to deal with the complex ethical, moral, legal, and medical issues during a disaster [15].

## References

[1] Wise G. Preparing for disaster: a way of developing community relationships. Disaster Manag Response 2006;5(1):14–7.

[2] Kennedy M. The Gulf Coast devastation: nurses respond to Hurricane Katrina. Am J Nurs 2005; 105(10):19.

[3] Volunteer worker page. Available at: http://www.redcross.org/services/volunteer/0,1082,0_325_,00.html. Accessed February 5, 2007.

[4] Hurricane Katrina Health Care Professionals and Relief Workers page. Available at http://www.hhs.gov/emergency/index.shtml. Accessed February 5, 2007.

[5] Health care professionals and relief personnel worker page, 2005. Available at: http://volunteer.ccrf.hhs.gov/. Accessed February 5, 2007.

[6] Marshall M. San Antonio mental health disaster consortium: Hurricanes Katrina and Rita, a personal perspective. Perspect Psychiatr Care 2007;43(1): 15–21.

[7] Senate Report 109–322—Hurricane Katrina: a nation still unprepared. Available at: http://www.gpoaccess.gov/serialset/creports/pdf/sr109/322/findings. Accessed June 29, 2007.

[8] McMahon M. The many codes for a disaster: a plea for standardization. Disaster Manag Response 2007;5:1–2.

[9] Cranmer H. Hurricane Katrina: volunteer work—logistics first. N Engl J Med 2005;353:1542–4.

[10] John P, Russell S, Russell P. The prevalence of post-traumatic stress disorder among children and adolescents affected by tsunami disaster in Tamil Nadu. Disaster Manag Response 2007;5:3–7.

[11] Mori K, Ugai K, Nonami Y, et al. Health needs of patients with chronic diseases who lived through the Great Hanshin earthquake. Disaster Manag Response 2007;5:8–13.

[12] Berggren R, Curiel T. After the storm—health care infrastructure in post-Katrina New Orleans. N Engl J Med 2006;354(15):1549–50.

[13] Clements PT, Garzon L, Milliken TF. Survivors' guilt following sudden traumatic loss: promoting early intervention in the critical care setting. Crit Care Nurs Clin North Am 2006;18:359–69.

[14] Berggren R. Hurricane Katrina: unexpected necessities-inside charity hospital. N Engl J Med 2005;353(15):1550–3.

[15] Curiel T. Murder or mercy? Hurricane Katrina and the need for disaster training. N Engl J Med 2006;355:2067–9.

[16] Henderson G. Finding supplies. N Engl J Med 2005;353(15):1543.

[17] Frohlich E. Aftershocks. N Engl J Med 2005;353(15):1545.

[18] Berger E. Charity hospital and disaster preparedness. Ann Emerg Med 2006;47(1):53–6.

[19] Greenough P, Kirsch T. Hurricane Katrina: public health response-assessing needs. N Engl J Med 2005;353:1544–6.

[20] Quick reference guide for the National Response Plan, Department of Homeland Security, version 4.0, 2006. Available at: http://www.dhs.gov/xlibrary/assets/NRP Quick_Reference_Guide_5-22-06.pdf. Accessed March 5, 2007.

[21] Berman M, Lazar E. Hospital emergency preparedness: lessons learned since Northridge. N Engl J Med 2003;348:1307–8.

[22] Vinson E. Managing bioterrorism mass casualties in an emergency department: lessons learned from a rural community hospital disaster drill. Disaster Manag Response 2007;5:18–21.

[23] Bioterrorism and other public health emergencies: altered standards of care in mass casualty events. Agency for Healthcare Research and Quality, United States Department of Health and Human Services. 2005. Available at: http://www.ahrq.gov/research/altstand/. Accessed January 11, 2007.

[24] American Nurses Association. ANA comments on nursing care 2006. Available at: http://nursingworld.org/PRESSREL/2006/PR092706.htm. Accessed February 13, 2007.

[25] Davies K, Hannigan C. Supporting disaster healthcare professionals: a practical and virtual approach. Nurse Educ Today 2006;27:122–30.

[26] McMahon M. Who will respond the next time? Disaster Manag Response 2006;4(4):97–8.

[27] Rhoads J, Mitchell F, Rick S. Posttraumatic stress disorder after Hurricane Katrina. JNP 2006;2(1):18–26.

[28] Traumatic incident stress: information for emergency response workers. Available at: http://www.cdc.gov/niosh/unp-trinstrs.html. Accessed April 7, 2007.

[29] Gaylord K. The psychosocial effects of combat: the frequently unseen injury. Crit Care Nurs Clin North Am 2006;18:349–57.

[30] McNally R. Psychological debriefing does not prevent posttraumatic stress disorder. Psychiatric Times 2004; Available at: http://www.psychiatrictimes.com/p040471.html Accessed March 4, 2007.

[31] Everly G, Flannery R, Eyler V. Critical incident stress management (CISM): a statistical review of the literature. Psychiatr Q 2002;73(3):171–82.

[32] Hammond J, Brooks J. The World Trade Center attack helping the helpers: the role of critical incident stress management. Crit Care 2001;5:315–7.

[33] Nieburg P, Waldman R, Krumm D. Evacuated populations-lessons from foreign refugee crises. N Engl J Med 2005;354(15):1547–9.

ELSEVIER
SAUNDERS

Crit Care Nurs Clin N Am 20 (2008) 91–102

CRITICAL CARE
NURSING CLINICS
OF NORTH AMERICA

# Managing a Disaster Scene and Multiple Casualties Before Help Arrives

## Janet Fraser Hale, PhD, APRN-BC, FNP, COL, AN, USAR (Ret)

*Graduate School of Nursing, University of Massachusetts,*
*55 Lake Avenue North, Worcester, MA 01655, USA*

A catastrophic event that can create significant human, structural, economic, and political devastation is generally described as a "high-impact event." These events include terrorist attacks with agents of terrorism (eg, chemical, biologic, radiologic, nuclear, and highly explosive devices), emerging or re-emerging infectious diseases, natural disasters, and accidental disasters. Recent examples of natural disasters are the 2004 tsunami in Southeast Asia, the ravages of Hurricanes Katrina and Rita on the Gulf Coast of the United States in 2005, and the 2007 tornados in central Florida, Alabama, and Kansas. Accidental disasters include a spill of hazardous materials, a chemical plant explosion, and airplane or train accidents. Citizens often think that manmade events occur only in larger cities, where the largest possible number of casualties would be inflicted, or where there are many important individuals whose death or injuries will have the most economic, political, or emotional impact. The reality is that terrorist events can occur at any place and any time; worse yet, multiple events could occur simultaneously around the country as on September 11, 2001 and as in other places, such as Israel, Iraq, and London.

As the largest group of health care professionals in the United States and a component of almost every community, nurses may be called upon to initiate the emergency response and provide initial planning for health care until local, regional, or federal assistance arrives. Even in communities with the best of public health planning, nurses may be the sole health care survivors after a high-impact event and/or the highest level of community health planner able to manage the scene and arrange for the care of injured victims. Such a scenario could result if community leaders were targeted or simply because of the sheer number of nurses. Consequently, it is important for nurses to understand the logistics of managing both the disaster scene and patient care in a disaster. Nurses also may report to a disaster as part of a team of responders in which they assume the traditional nursing role (ie, providing one-on-one care to victims under the guidance of physicians). Whether a nurse responds in a traditional nursing role or is the most prepared professional available during the initial management of the scene and is being pushed to extremes of scope of practice and beyond, it is important to have a sense of the greater picture of disaster management. It is imperative to understand why those in charge may be making decisions and contingency plans that seem counterintuitive. For example, care could be directed first to those least injured, seemingly sick patients might be evacuated from hospitals and nursing homes, or the 3-day weather forecast might be a pressing concern.

Preparedness for bioterrorism has been well addressed in the literature [1–5], especially since the anthrax events in Washington DC, Florida, and Connecticut following September 11, 2001. The response to and management of all types of disasters, in addition to bioterrorism, have many commonalities that can be applied to any event

The views expressed in this manuscript are those of the author and do not reflect the official policy or position of the Department of the Army, Department of Defense, or the United States Government.

*E-mail address:* janet.hale@umassmed.edu

0899-5885/08/$ - see front matter. Published by Elsevier Inc.
doi:10.1016/j.ccell.2007.10.012

*ccnursing.theclinics.com*

in which casualties exceed the capabilities of a health care system. As the potential for and complexity of high-impact events evolves, health care professionals, and particularly nurses, clearly need a general template for all-hazards preparedness and response to any high-impact event.

The purpose of this article is to increase nurses' ability to anticipate, prepare for, and respond to multi-casualty, high-impact events. Empowered with this information, nurses will have tools to manage the disaster scene until help arrives from emergency medical services, the public health department, and other local, state, and possibly federal agencies. Resources for more in-depth information on prevention, preparedness and planning, and the health systems' response are included. The article concludes with the emotionally charged consideration of triaging multi-casualties in the face of scarce resources.

With international tensions continuously at a high level, additional successful high-impact events are possible in the United States. Americans were stunned in 2001 when commercial airplanes were hijacked and used as highly explosive devices to damage significant political, economic, and historic landmarks in the United States. A sobering article written in 2004 suggests that the United States could begin to experience terrorist tactics similar to the suicide bombing campaign in Israel [6]. Furthermore, the question of pandemic influenza striking the United States is not if it will occur, but when [7].

Given these dangers, nurses can be empowered by having considered some scenarios that these disasters are likely to create. Armed with the appropriate knowledge, nurses will be prepared if they find themselves the most informed professional at a scene. They will be able to manage the scene within the constraints of available resources. They must be able to think quickly, improvise, teach and delegate, and manage until help arrives. As Hurricane Katrina showed, the arrival of help (eg, emergency medical services, public health personnel, and/or federal assistance) could be delayed for hours, days, or even weeks. In the case of simultaneous events occurring across the country, it could be much longer before the authorities can provide relief.

## Preparedness

The more prepared a nurse is for a high-impact event, the better is his/her ability to respond. Preparation involves planning at the individual,

community, and professional level. Planning starts with preparing oneself, assessing the surrounding community for its risks and vulnerabilities, and preparing professionally to be a knowledgeable responder.

### Personal preparation

Everyone should be personally prepared for an emergency. Health professionals should not respond to any emergency or disaster event unless they are prepared at home and have a plan for the care of family, children, and pets should they need to be away for a long period. This absence could be voluntary or required. For example, one could deploy voluntarily to another community in response to a disaster. A nurse also could be mandated by his/her institution to deploy or could be quarantined if the institution houses a patient with a highly infectious disease. The bottom line is that nurses need to be personally prepared at home, so that they are not distracted on the job with concerns about what is happening at home. All families should be prepared to shelter in place, meaning to take immediate shelter wherever they are (eg, home, work, or school).

There is no consensus on whether families should be prepared for 3 days [8], 2 weeks [9,10], or longer [11], but all homes should have a minimum of 3 days of supplies that include high-protein, nonperishable, ready-to-eat canned foods (with a manual can opener), water (1 gallon per person per day), medications (prescription and nonprescription), waterproof matches, candles, flashlights with extra batteries, first-aid kit, a battery-operated radio with extra batteries, extra toilet paper, bleach, feminine supplies, glasses, contact lens solution, basic tools (eg, hammer, wrench, screwdriver, pliers), duct tape, plastic sheeting, various sizes of plastic bags, pet supplies, copies of important phone numbers, and important papers [8–11]. Some families have even purchased generators to provide power in case of a massive power outage.

Supplies should be stored in a specific place where they can be readily located and even packed if evacuation is necessary. Given that items such as medications and water have expiration dates, emergency supplies should be rotated routinely to ensure they are always fresh.

### Community preparation

In the current world order, or disorder, everyone must be vigilant and aware of their surroundings. No one can afford to be complacent! Nurses must understand the possible risks and vulnerabilities inherent in their own community. Terrorists seek targets that are symbolically significant and will inflict mass casualties. They want to weaken the human spirit and create fear in United States citizens with the threat of massive violence and bloodshed.

In thinking about a possible high-impact event in one's own community, one must assess the likelihood of natural disasters and potential terrorist targets in the area. Most people understand their community's risk for natural disasters such as earthquakes, droughts, floods, hurricanes, or tornadoes, but they may not have considered the potential for terrorist events. Terrorist targets might include nuclear power plants, dams, generating facilities, fuel farms, refineries, pipelines, hazardous materials freight, financial institutions, government buildings, symbolic buildings and monuments, and civil aviation. People could be specifically targeted at political conventions and other large gatherings of people (eg, rock concerts and highly visible sporting events such as the Super Bowl). More common targets could include gas stations, subways, trains, bridges, and tunnels.

*Professional preparation*

Nurses should not become "spontaneous unaffiliated volunteers," who create problems during a disaster [12]. In response to Hurricanes Katrina and Rita, many health care volunteers traveled long distances, at their own expense, to the Gulf Coast. Despite their well-meaning intentions, however, many of these volunteers were not enthusiastically welcomed, and, worse yet, some were sent home without having an opportunity to contribute at all. Volunteers need to be formally and nationally credentialed. They need to understand their role, responsibilities, and the chain of command and communication. Volunteers who show up without being officially credentialed will not be used at all or will serve at a level far below their capabilities and professional expertise. Showing original license(s) and certifications does not help.

Professional preparation begins with understanding one's state rules and regulations on prescribed professional responsibilities, volunteering, and/or required participation in an institutional or community disaster. Nurses must understand the emergency preparedness plan for their employing institution and their role, if any,

in that plan. They should seek opportunities to be involved with the emergency and disaster-planning initiatives for their institution so that they will be involved in the drills and become familiar with the strengths and weaknesses of the plan. Participating in these drills increases communication and builds relationships among the community entities involved in an emergency response. Beyond that, nurses can consider state and national registries designed to contribute to the United States' surge capacity by increasing the number of available, nationally credentialed health care professionals to meet current and future health care needs resulting from a high-impact event [13].

Nurses are cautioned to register officially with only one national registry; otherwise they will be counted as an asset by all those with whom they have registered. In fact, nurses can deploy with only one registry should the need arise, and the other agencies no longer have an asset on which they had counted [13]. Nurses should inform their employing institution of this registration. Most registries expect that nurses understand their own institution's emergency and disaster plan, the facility's expectations of employees during an emergency event, and the nurse's role in such an event.

For registered nurses who volunteer for disasters, two work-release guidelines have been developed [14,15]. One includes the rights and responsibilities of the nurse [14], and the other provides a guide for employers [15]. Volunteer health professionals probably will have a better environment during emergency events because of uniform state legislation being developed by the American Nurses Association and the National Conference of Commissioners on Uniform State Laws. Under consideration is a Uniform Emergency Volunteer Health Care Practitioners Act, with final action expected in the near future [13].

*Registered volunteer options*

Four national registered volunteer programs are presented in Table 1: Emergency System for Advance Registration of Volunteer Health Professionals (ESAR-VHP), Medical Reserve Corps (MRC), Disaster Medical Assistance Teams (DMAT), and the American Red Cross. Nurses who register with one of these organizations should inform their employing institution of the volunteer program, the degree of deployment for which they have volunteered (ie, for local mass

Table 1
Registered volunteer options

| Name | Type of organization | Expectations/requirements | Range of deployability |
|---|---|---|---|
| Emergency System for Advance Registration of Volunteer Health Professionals (ESAR-VHP) | State-based electronic database of health care personnel (at all levels and disciplines) Registers volunteers, verifies their credentials and qualifications for an emergency Funded and overseen by the Health Resources and Systems Administration | This program and has on-line training requirements related to the federally supported Incident Command System (ICS) that must be completed before applicants are fully registered. | Facilitates states' ability to identify and use health professional volunteers in emergencies and disasters. This system will allow professionals to cross state lines to participate in a disaster response if needed [13,16,17]. |
| Medical Reserve Corps (MRC) | Incorporates interdisciplinary groups of local medical and public health professionals who volunteer their time and expertise to prepare for and respond to emergencies, thus supplementing official emergency and public health resources. | National MRC office comes under the Office of the US Surgeon General. MRC units are organized and managed at the community level [13,18]. Preparation varies by communities. | Community based and focused. |
| Disaster Medical Assistance Teams (DMAT) | DMATs are part of the National Disaster Medical System (NDMS). | Consists of well-prepared, organized, and trained teams of health care professionals available to maintain a national capability to deliver quality medical care to the victims of and responders to a domestic disaster [19] | Most likely to be prepared to respond and/or be deployed nationally in case of need. |
| American Red Cross | The American Red Cross is a humanitarian organization that provides relief to victims of disasters [20]. | Specialized training to prevent, prepare for, and respond to for disasters. | Can deploy to national or international emergencies. |

immunizations only, local community responses only, state, national, or even international deployment), and how the deployment might affect their availability for staffing their own institution. The application forms for these programs address deployment interest and the volunteer's willingness to go outside the community, the state, and in some cases the country. Nurse volunteers would be prudent to check if their personal liability and/or professional insurance, if any, cover actions taken during a disaster and/or if the disaster relief organization provides insurance for volunteers.

## Health systems' response

All high-impact events begin as local disasters. When an event creates health care demands that overwhelm a community's resources, community leaders initiate a chain of requests for help. These local leaders (eg, health department officials, mayor, or law enforcement) call on state officials (eg, state health department, governor, or the National Guard), who ultimately may request help at the national level. If the event is considered an incident of national significance that requires a coordinated federal response, the National Response Plan is invoked.

The National Response Plan has two key components: the Incident Command System (ICS) and the National Incident Management System (NIMS). The ICS ensures consistency and interagency communication, understanding, and cooperation by serving as the primary framework for managing events. The ICS is a well-known management concept already practiced by hazardous-material teams, firefighters, rescuers, and emergency response teams. This system standardizes the management of all hazards at all government levels by using common terms and by identifying specific positions and job descriptions for event management and communication [21]. The NIMS, which can be considered the "ICS of the national level," is called into play when a high-impact event requires a coordinated national response with interagency communication and collaboration. The NIMS, which is administered by the Federal Emergency Management Agency (FEMA), was created to improve coordination among responders from different jurisdictions and disciplines. The NIMS offers a unified approach to incident management and standard command and management structures and emphasizes preparedness, mutual aid, and resource management [22].

Understanding the structure of the ICS and the NIMS is helpful for responders. Also, this knowledge is part of the short on-line courses required to credential volunteers to organizations such as the ESAR-VHP and the MRC. The Hospital Incident Command System (HICS), which is the hospital-level version of the ICS, is widely used by hospitals in their disaster plans for establishing emergency operations centers [23]. As such, the HICS fits hand-in-glove with the higher levels of ICS and the NIMS structure, allowing consistency, continuity, and communication between and among agencies and organizations at all levels. These relationships and communication using common terms and processes are vital to the success of any disaster response. In summary, an emergency in a hospital would invoke the HICS; if the whole community were involved, the ICS would be involved to manage all the community's hospitals and other agencies in their response. If an event becomes an incident of national interest, the NIMS would be called into play as part of the overall National Response Plan.

## Potential for leadership

Nurses are highly respected and trusted by the public as informed and trained professionals.

During an emergency, most citizens will look to nurses for guidance, assistance, and care. Nurses can be empowered for this role by educating themselves to make significant contributions to preserving life and to leading the emergency management initiative, if needed, until help arrives.

To guide registered nurses toward maximizing their potential contributions during a mass casualty event, the Nursing Emergency Preparedness Education Coalition (previously known as the International Nursing Coalition for Mass Casualty Education) released a set of 63 competencies for entry-level registered nurses to handle mass casualty incidents [24]. These competencies are organized under four core competencies (ie, critical thinking, assessment, technical skills, communication), six core knowledge areas (ie, 1) health promotion, risk reduction, and disease prevention, 2) health care systems and policy, 3) illness and disease management, 4) information and health care technologies, 5) ethics, and 6) human diversity), and the last section of the competencies addresses professional role development [24]. To meet these competencies, nurses can use interactive, on-line modules developed by the National Nurse Emergency Preparedness Initiative to learn about the various agents of terrorism, how to respond in a disaster, and how to manage patients [25]. These modules will be released in the near future with free access, including continuing education units at no cost.

Furthermore, a national panel of Advanced Practice Registered Nurse stakeholders, sponsored by the National Organization for Nurse Practitioner Faculties and supported by the National Nurse Emergency Preparedness Initiative, has prepared a document to be used as a guide by advanced practice nursing programs when considering program content related to emergency preparedness and all-hazards response to high-impact events [26]. The content and resources have been organized around 11 competencies [27,28] currently used by the Health Resources and Services Administration (HRSA) to evaluate 26 HRSA-funded Bioterrorism Training and Curriculum Development Program sites [29]. The final document is offered for program consideration but is not meant to be prescriptive [26].

Nurses are encouraged to take advantage of these learning opportunities to prepare themselves for care situations about which they may not have been previously educated. Additionally, core disaster life-support, basic disaster life-support, and advanced disaster life-support courses are available through universities and organizations, such as the Medical College of Georgia, the University of Alabama Birmingham, the American Medical Association, and the Wisconsin Medical Society. Nurses who participate in disaster-preparedness education and simulated exercises have more knowledge and ability for a comprehensive response to emergencies, and therefore are more likely to recognize a potential event and to implement appropriate leadership behaviors, than those who have not done so [4].

### Be Safe!

To be good clinicians and good leaders at an emergency scene, nurses must remember to protect themselves first. One will not be much help if he/she becomes a victim, so personal safety and protection must be considered before rushing in to respond. For example, if a responder is exposed to a virulent agent or contaminated with a hazardous chemical, he/she may not be allowed to leave the area to go home for an indeterminate period. In such a case, the clinician would no longer be available to help but instead would need help from another provider. Thus, it is prudent for nurses to know and understand how to protect themselves and how to wear personal protective equipment as needed and when available.

### Managing the scene

Health care professionals who arrive at the scene of a disaster generally think first and foremost of caring for the victims. Before taking on this complex and ethically challenging task, which is discussed in the next section, nurses need to consider the larger context of scene management. Thus, this section discusses mapping the disaster area, plotting weather patterns, caring for caregivers, securing hospitals, creating surge capacity, and activating the Strategic National Stockpile.

### Mapping the disaster area

In scene management, many decisions and plans must come together in a relatively short time. To facilitate this process, a large and detailed wall-mounted map of the local area will be invaluable. If such a map is not available, it may need to be sketched by hand until an accurate map can be obtained from the local health department or Internet. This map should be used to plot the major roads (evacuation routes), health care facilities (functioning and non-functioning), and possible alternate sites of care to turn victims into patients. It also is important to identify health care facilities that may be damaged and/or no longer in use, as well as roads that are damaged and inaccessible, contaminated areas, and damaged infrastructures throughout the area. This information will help in determining the routes and destinations for transporting victims for definitive care as quickly as possible.

### Plotting weather patterns

Because a high-impact event will be influenced by weather conditions, weather patterns should be overlaid on the map to show wind drift, present and future temperatures, precipitation, and other details. The potency and durability of released aerosolized terrorist agents would be affected significantly by precipitation, wind, and temperature. Plotting wind direction also would identify additional affected or contaminated areas downwind of the initial blast, explosion, or release of an agent. The weather also will affect victims and rescuers greatly. Cold temperatures increase the risk of hypothermia. Heat, especially when combined with humidity, increases the risk of dehydration, in turn increasing the need for planned rest periods throughout rescuers' shifts and for potable water and nourishment. The weather also can contribute to difficulties in transport (eg, snow, ice) and air evacuation (eg, heavy winds, low cloud ceiling, fog, or rain).

### Caring for caregivers

The rescuers/responders will need to be monitored closely to ensure that they are supplied with the necessary, food, water, shelter, and rest as dictated by the duration of the response. Ensuring adequate levels of respite/backup personnel and supplies should begin early in the emergency response to avoid being caught short, and plans should be made immediately for replenishing these supplies as the days and the scene progress over time. For any high-impact event with a prolonged response, shift rotations should begin immediately, to avoid burning out and exhausting all rescuers/responders in the first few hours.

### Securing hospitals

All hospitals will need to evaluate the need for additional security and a plan for controlled entry. When people panic and fear for their health and safety, they are likely to seek care at a hospital. Large numbers of victims/patients will overwhelm a hospital's available assets to provide care. At facilities with multiple entrances, thought should be given early on to ensuring that only one entrance is operational for entry and exit. This step will allow administrators to monitor the numbers of employees, volunteers, and others entering and to manage the entrance of patients and other concerned citizens. This precaution becomes particularly important to contain patients, visitors, and/or health care professionals infected with or exposed to a highly infectious, deadly agent. Similarly, restricting access will help manage the huge influx of contaminated or exposed victims from outside the facility who may attempt to swarm entrances for care. Although such a move is a very difficult decision to make and a difficult feat to accomplish, it will be necessary, because even one contaminated person gaining entrance could contaminate the entire facility in short order. Clearly, instances such as these depict how important good communication and good relationships with law enforcement and emergency medical services will be to the protection and safety of all.

*Creating surge capacity*

Creating surge capacity within the health care system involves making decisions at several levels. The first step is to cancel all nonessential admissions and surgeries and to discharge all patients who could be cared for at home or at a lower level of care (eg, nursing home, rehabilitation facility, or alternate care site). Evacuation of hospitals and nursing homes must be considered to make room for large numbers of seriously injured victims. The next step is to consider how these patients will be transported from point A to point B (eg, from a hospital to a nursing home, from a nursing home to a home or to an alternate care site). Nurses may also be instrumental in planning for and staffing alternate sites of care in school gymnasiums, armories, and other large warehouse-type facilities. In developing alternate sites of care, planners should consider the availability of running potable water and electricity in any facility used for patient care.

Within hospitals, which will be the destination of most seriously injured/ill victims, operating rooms may need to be staffed and functioning around the clock if an event results in a large number of traumatic injuries requiring surgery. Depending on the type of event, units may need to change their scope to burn patients (explosion), ventilator-assisted patients (botulism, plague), or isolation (anthrax, plague, viral hemorrhagic fevers, small pox). If blood products for transfusions are in short supply, healthy rescuers and providers should be considered for blood donations until additional blood and blood products can be procured.

*Activating the Strategic National Stockpile*

If an event seems likely to become long lasting, and available resources are depleting rapidly, the Strategic National Stockpile can be activated federally to release pharmaceuticals (eg, antibiotics, chemical antidotes, antitoxins, life-support medications) and medical supplies (eg, intravenous administration supplies, airway maintenance supplies, and medical/surgical items) at no charge. Within 12 hours of the initial request, these items, already packed in huge Plexiglas containers, can be transported to any state. The Strategic National Stockpile is designed to resupply state and local public health agencies in the event of a national emergency anywhere within the United States or its territories. The request is made from the local level up through the chain-of-command system of the city, county, and state, to the federal level [30].

**Managing victims at the scene**

Managing the care of victim/patients during a high-impact event presents numerous challenges, including an uncertain physical environment, personal risk (as discussed previously), and limited health care personnel and medical resources [13]. In anticipating how to manage mass casualties in a community, one must think about those who populate it. Does the community have predominantly older families or retirees who may have multiple comorbidities, increased disabilities, and less responsive immune systems? Is it a bedroom community of working parents, many children, schools, and childcare facilities? Is it a community of many universities and colleges with a population of young adults and older adolescents? The populations to be served will determine the issues and challenges that may be encountered as well as the specialty health care professionals that may be needed (eg, geriatricians, pediatricians, or obstetricians). The need for and importance of pastoral care and mental health assistance cannot be underestimated in any high-impact event.

*Standard triage*

As potential first responders to an incident, nurses should have a basic understanding of triage. Hospital emergency departments use essentially three major triage categories or some variant thereof: (1) emergent, (2) urgent, and (3) nonurgent. "Emergent," the common triage term for emergency cases, are cases needing immediate (within 10 or 20 minutes) resuscitation/treatment efforts for survival. Urgent cases require care within 2 hours, and those with nonurgent/minor illness or injury can wait safely longer than 2 hours. Regardless of the triage system, the sickest/most-injured patients are seen first. Rarely, if ever, is consideration given to how many resources may be needed or consumed in resuscitation efforts to salvage/sustain life. The triage nurse's duty is to reassess waiting patients continually for any change in their condition that might move them up on the priority list.

*Multiple-casualty triage*

Situations that create casualties in numbers far exceeding the available resources and supplies, whether in- or outside an emergency department, will call for a different system of triage. Rather than identifying the sickest or most-injured patients and caring for them first, field triage from a high-impact event requires a quick initial assessment and categorization of victims so that, as additional help arrives, responders can be directed easily to those most in need of attention. The general approach is to separate those who are likely to do well with delayed care, those needing immediate life-saving care that can be done quickly with few resources, those minimally injured who are able to care for themselves and help others, and those who are likely to die without heroic measures and consumption of scarce resources [31–36]. See Table 2 for the categories for mass casualty triage, identification, and color coding.

One easy, practical system for initially sorting people at a disaster site into relatively meaningful categories is first to invite everyone who can hear the announcement and can walk to move to a specific area such as a bus, field, or parking lot. Depending on their injuries, these persons may be able to assist the rescuers (eg, by staying with and comforting patients in need, bringing supplies, or holding pressure on a bleeding wound). Next, ask everyone who can hear the announcement but cannot walk or move to another area to raise or wave their hands. These persons should be assessed and treated quickly, (eg, by opening an airway, applying a tourniquet to a spurting artery, or putting an occlusive dressing on a sucking chest wound). Patients can be tagged by color indicating their triage category to help later arriving professionals identify where they should focus their efforts (see Table 2).

Finally, those who do not respond by raising their hands or motioning in some way are initially considered expectant (dead or expected to die), and their treatment should be delayed. "Expectant" is a term often used in mass casualty triage (situations in which the number of victims exceeds the capacity of the health care system) to indicate those who probably will die without protracted resuscitation efforts. Such efforts would consume large amounts of medical resources, including personnel, at the expense of saving many other victims needing fewer resources and immediate, but short-term resuscitation efforts. The expectant group should be provided palliative care until additional personnel and/or resources arrive to reassess their health status and medical needs. The terminal or expectant group should never be left unattended. Their needs should be met by pastoral and mental health volunteers. Morphine and other pain-relieving medications should be used liberally, and palliative care should be a standard treatment. In a catastrophic event creating mass casualties, not all patients can be saved, but the goal is to save as many as possible.

Table 2
Categories for mass casualty triage, identification, and color tagging

| Category | Action | Color code | Treatment |
|----------|--------|------------|-----------|
| Minor | Delayed care | Green | Can delay up to 3 hours |
| Delayed | Urgent care | Yellow | Can delay up to 1 hour |
| Immediate | Immediate care | Red | Life-threatening |
| Expectant | Multiple injuries/trauma, terminal illness, fatal injuries | Black | Palliative care for patients and families |
| Deceased | Morgue/refrigeration until further options available | Black | Dignified care of the remains |

*Data from* Simple Triage and Rapid Treatment (START). Available at: http://www.citmt.org/start/background. htm. Accessed April 11, 2007; and Basic disaster life support. Available at: http://www.emhelpcenter.org/bdls_information. html. Accessed April 30, 2007.

**Box 1. Sources of further information**

- Aeromedical evacuation. Available at: http://navymedicine.med.navy.mil/Files/Media/directives/5115.pdf
- Altered Standards of Care in Mass Casualty Events. Available at: http://www.ahrq.gov/research/mce/
- Bioterrorism and Other Public Health Emergencies Tools and Models for Planning and Preparedness. Cantrill SV. National Hospital Available Beds for Emergencies and Disasters (HAvBED) System: Final Report. Available at: http://www.ahrq.gov/research/havbed
- Bioterrorism and Emergency Preparedness Program. Available at: http://www.ahrq.gov/path/biotrspn.htm
- Centers for Disease Control: Emergency Preparedness and Response: Agents, Disease, & Other Threats—Bioterrorism, Chemical Emergencies, Radiation Emergencies, Mass Casualties, Natural Disasters & Severe Weather, Recent Outbreaks & Incidents, Available at: http://www.bt.cdc.gov/
- Control of Communicable Diseases in Man. 18th edition. Heymann DL, editor. Washington (DC): American Public Health Association; 2004
- Development of Models for Emergency Preparedness: Personal Protective Equipment, Decontamination, Isolation/Quarantine, and Laboratory Capacity: PPE Classifications. Available at: www.ahrq.gov/research/devmodels/devmodel2a.htm
- Emergency Risk Communication for Public Health Professionals. Available at: http://www.nwcphp.org/edu/training/courses-exercises/courses/risk-communication
- FEMA Independent Study Program: A National Response Plan, An Introduction. Available at: http://www.training.fema.gov/emiweb/IS/is800a.asp

- HANDBOOKS (available at: https://ccc.apgea.army.mil/products/handbooks/books.htm)
  - *Field Management of Chemical Casualties*
  - Medical Management of Chemical Casualties—The Red Book
  - Medical Management of Biological Casualties—The Blue Book
  - Medical Management of Radiological Casualties
  - The Medical NBC Battle Book.
- Treatment of Biological Warfare Agent Casualties—Field Manual
  - Biologic-induced illness—pocket card
  - Radiation-induced illness—pocket card
  - Chemical-induced illness—pocket card
  - Blasts and explosions—pocket card
- HAZMAT: Emergency Response Guide. Available at: http://hazmat.dot.gov/pubs/erg/gydebook.htm
- Hospital Incident Command System. Available at: http://www.emsa.ca.gov/dms2/heics_hics.pdf
- Incident Command. Available at: http://www.training.fema.gov/EMIWeb/IS/ICSResource/index.htm
- Joint Commission on Accreditation of Healthcare Organizations Emergency Management Standards. Handbook of Bioterrorism and Disaster Medicine. 2006. Available at: www.springerlink.com/content/j413881268uu1130/
- Joint Commission Guide to Emergency Management Planning in Health Care. Available at: www.jcrinc.com/1022
- Lessons learned in information systems. Available at: http://www.llis.gov
- Mass Medical Care with Scarce Resources: A Community Planning Guide. Available at: www.ahrq.gov/research/mce/mceguide.pdf
- Mental Health All-Hazards Disaster Planning Guidance. Available at: http://mentalhealth.samhsa.gov/

disasterrelief/publications/allpubs/
SMA03-3829/part_four.asp
- National Incident Management
  System. Available at: http://
  www.nimsonline.com/
- National Infrastructure Protection Plan:
  Sector Overview. Available at: http://
  www.dhs.gov/xlibrary/assets/
  NIPP_SectorOverview.pdf
- National Response Plan. Available at:
  http://www.dhs.gov/xprepresp/
  committees/editorial_0566.shtm
- NIOSH Safety and Health Topic:
  Emergency Response Resources.
  Available at: *www.ahrq.gov/research/
  devmodels/devmodel2a.htm*
- OSHA Best Practices for
  Hospital-Based First Receivers of
  Victims. Available at: http://www.osha.
  gov/dts/osta/bestpractices/
  firstreceivers_hospital.html
- Pandemic Influenza. Available at:
  http://www.pandemicflu.gov
- Pediatric Terrorism and Disaster
  Preparedness: A Resource for
  Pediatricians. AHRQ Publication Nos.
  06(07)-0056 and 06(07)-0056-1.
  Rockville (MD): Agency for Health care
  Research and Quality; 2006: Available
  at: http://.ahrq.gov/research/pedpre/
  resource.htm
- Preparing for the Psychological
  Consequences of Terrorism: A Public
  Health Strategy (2003). Available at:
  http://books.nap.edu/
  openbook.php?isbn=0,309,089,530
- Providing Medical Care with Scarce
  Resources: Strategies and Tools for
  Community Planners. Available at:
  http://www.ahrq.gov/research/mce
- Radiation
  Radiation basics. Available at: http://
    www.orau.gov/reacts/define.htm/
  Radiation Emergencies. Available at:
    http://www.bt.cdc.gov/radiation/
  Managing radiation emergencies.
    Available at: http://www.orau.gov/
    reacts/procedures.htm
  Hospital Triage in the First 24 Hours
    after a Nuclear or Radiological
    Incident. Available at: http://
    www.orau.gov/reacts/triage.pdf

Acute radiation syndrome. Available
  at: http://www.bt.cdc.gov/radiation/
  arsphysicianfactsheet.asp
Prenatal radiation exposure: a fact
  sheet for physicians. Available at:
  http://www.bt.cdc.gov/radiation/
  prenatalphysician.asp
Software to record radiological
  incidents and assess dose rates.
  Available at: http://
  www.afrri.usuhs.mil/
Terrorism with ionizing radiation
  general guidance: pocket guide.
  Available at: http://
  www.afrri.usuhs.mil/www/outreach/
  pdf/pcktcard.pdf
- Simple Triage and Rapid Treatment
  (START). The START system relies on
  rapidly (< 1 minute) assessing patients,
  determining in which of four
  categories patients fall, and visibly
  labeling categories for rescuers who
  will treat patients. Available at: http://
  www.citmt.org/start/background.htm
- State Department of Public Health
  Website and resources. Available at:
  http://www.statepublichealth.org
- Surge Capacity: CDC Mass Casualties:
  In a Moment's Notice: Surge capacity
  in terrorist bombings–Challenges and
  Proposed Solutions. Available at:
  http://www.bt.cdc.gov/masscasualties/
  surgecapacity.asp
- Taking Care of Yourself …. Field
  Hygiene and Sanitation. Available at:
  http://chppm-www.apgea.army.mil/
  deployment/fm21-10.pdf
- The JumpSTART Pediatric MCI Triage
  Tool and other pediatric disaster and
  emergency medicine resources.
  Available at: http://
  www.jumpstarttriage.com/
  JumpSTART_and_MCI_Triage.php
- Tips for Managing and Preventing
  Stress: A Guide for Emergency and
  Disaster Response Workers. Available
  at: http://mentalhealth.samhsa.gov/
  publications/allpubs/KEN-01-0098/
- Urban Institute report on Katrina.
  Available at: http://www.urban.org/
  afterkatrina/

- White Ribbon Alliance, Women and Infants Service Package (WISP) of the White Ribbon Alliance for Safe Motherhood. National Working Group for Women and Infant Need in Emergencies. Available at: http://www.whiteribbonalliance.org/Resources/Documents/WISP

---

Note: This list is drawn from resources of state and federal government organizations and agencies that are likely to respond to high-impact events. It is important to use resources such as these, which are routinely reviewed, updated and revised as appropriate, because best practices may change in accordance with constantly changing evidence and lessons learned over time. Items are presented in alphabetical order, because most of the listed resources cover many topics associated with the content of this article.

*Data from* National Organization of Nurse Practitioner Faculties. APRN education for emergency preparedness and all hazards response: resources and suggested content; 2007. Available at: www.NONPF.com. Accessed November 17, 2007.

*Rationing scarce resources*

Ideally, communities would have prepared for the potential need to ration care by consulting with stakeholders and an ethicist and by holding open planning discussions on how to manage and ration resources if victims far outnumber the available health care personnel, supplies, and equipment. Because this issue involves significant ethical and moral decisions that are heavily laden with values and emotions, the more community stakeholders, faith-based leaders, and community representatives that can be involved in discussions and planning, the better and the more transparent the necessity, plans and process will be. During a high-impact event, in which a decision for rationing must be made and announced, the more transparent the process has been to the community, and especially to the media, the more acceptable it is likely to be to the community that will be so deeply affected [34,35]. When it is necessary to ration scarce resources (eg, vaccines, pandemic influenza treatments, and/or limited ventilators), values will be placed on human lives in determining the priorities. These decisions are

difficult and challenging, because the choice is never clear or easy. The Agency for Health Care Research and Quality has released its 2007 community-planning guide in the event of a mass disaster [35], and the American Nurses Association is in the final stages of releasing its review of nursing standards and guidelines during emergencies and disasters [34]. These guides address in more depth the difficulties and challenges faced during events resulting in multiple casualties.

**Summary**

This article presents an overview of common issues for nurses to consider when preparing for and responding to all types of high-impact events. Information was provided for nurses to begin preparing for the important leadership and management roles they may have to assume in such an event. The more informed and prepared nurses are, the easier it will be for them to assume these important roles as leaders or team members. More in-depth information for every area discussed can be found in the resources listed in Box 1 [26].

**Acknowledgments**

The author sincerely thanks Claire Baldwin, MS, for her quality, timely guidance and editorial suggestions in preparing the article.

**References**

[1] Biscup PJ, Gunther SD, Strawder AS, et al. Bioterrorism information handbook. Baltimore (MD): Veterans Affairs of MD Health Care System: Department of Pharmacy Services; 2002.

[2] Coleman EA. Emergency mass casualty: tularemia—a practical guide to management in the event of a tick bite or terrorist attack. Am J Nurs 2002;102(6):65–9.

[3] O'Brien KK, Higdon ML, Halverson JJ. Recognition and management of bioterrorism infections. Am Fam Physician 2003;67(9):1927–34.

[4] Rebmann T. Defining bioterrorism preparedness for nurses: concept analysis. J Adv Nurs 2006;54(5):623–32.

[5] Steed CJ, Howe L, Pruitt R, et al. Integrating bioterrorism education into nursing school curricula. J Nurs Educ 2006;43(8):362–7.

[6] Nunn S. Thinking the inevitable: suicide attacks in America and the design of effective public safety policies. Journal of Homeland Security and Emergency Management 2004;1(4): 401:18. Available at: http://www.bepress.com/jhsem/vol1/iss4/401. Accessed November 17, 2007.

[7] Barclay L. World Health Organization issues new guidelines for the avian flu virus. Lancet Infect Dis 2007;7:21–31.

[8] Ready America. Available at: http://www.ready.gov/america/getakit. Accessed April 28, 2007.

[9] CDC pandemic flu guidance. Available at: http://www.pandemicflu.gov/plan. Accessed April 28, 2007.

[10] Red Cross plan. Available at: http://www.redcross.org/news/ds/panflu/planahead.html. Accessed April 28, 2007.

[11] Latter Day Saints storage guidance. Available at: http://www.lds.about.com/library/weekly. Accessed April 28, 2007.

[12] Office of the Surgeon General. Pandemic influenza planning guidance for Medical Reserve Corps units. 2006; Available at: http://www.medicalreservecorps.gov/POUpdates/PandemicFluGuidance. Accessed April 16, 2007.

[13] Peterson CA. Be safe, be prepared: emergency system for advanced registration of volunteer health professionals in disaster response. Online J Issues Nurs 2006; 11(3). Available at: http://www.medscape.com/viewarticle/546009. Accessed November 17, 2007.

[14] American Nurses Association. Registered nurses' rights and responsibilities related to work release during a disaster. Available at: http://www.nursingworld.org/readroom/position/social. Accessed April 16, 2007.

[15] American Nurses Association. Work release during a disaster—guidelines for employers. Available at: http://www.nursingworld.org/readroom/position/social. Accessed April 16, 2007.

[16] US Department of Health and Human Services Health Resources and Systems Administration. Emergency system for advance registration of volunteer health professionals. Available at: http://www.hrsa.gov/esarvhp/. Accessed March 25, 2007.

[17] American Hospital Association. Emergency system for advanced registration of volunteer health care personnel—hospital implementation issues and solutions focus group meeting report 2005. Available at: www.hrsa.gov/esarvhp/FocusGroupReport0705/default.htm. Accessed April 16, 2007.

[18] Office of the Surgeon General. Medical Reserve Corps. Available at: http://www.medicalreservecorps.gov. Accessed March 25, 2007.

[19] National Defense Management System DMAT. Available at: http://www.oep-ndms.dhhs.gov/dmat.html. Accessed March 10, 2007.

[20] American Red Cross. Available at: http://www.redcross.org. Accessed March 10, 2007.

[21] Incident Command System. Available at: http://www.training.fema.gov/EMIWeb/IS/ICSResource/index.htm. Accessed April 9, 2007.

[22] National Incident Management System (NIMS). Available at: http://www.nimsonline.com. Accessed April 9, 2007.

[23] Hospital Emergency Incident Command System update. Available at: http://www.emsa.ca.gov/dms2/heics_hics.pdf. Accessed April 30, 2007.

[24] Stanley J. INCMCE Educational competencies for registered nurses responding to mass casualty incidents. July 2003. Available at: http://www.incmce.org/competenciespage.html. Accessed November 17, 2007.

[25] National Nurse Emergency Preparedness Initiative. Available at: http://www.nnepi.org. Accessed April 28, 2007.

[26] APRN education for emergency preparedness and all hazards response: resources and suggested content. Available at: www.NONPF.com. Accessed November 17, 2007.

[27] Gebbie KM, Qureshi K. Emergency and disaster preparedness: core competencies for nurses: what every nurse should but may not know. Am J Nurs 2002;102(1):46–51.

[28] Columbia University School of Nursing. Center for Health Policy. Clinician competencies during initial assessment and management of emergency events. Available at: http://sklad.cumc.columbia.edu/nursing/CHP/order Pubs.php. Accessed April 23, 2007.

[29] Health Resources and Services Administration. HRSA06N2345532SA Request for Task Order under Category I: characteristics of successful training for bioterrorism training and curriculum development. Available at: http://apply.grants.gov/opportunities/instructions/oppHRSA-06-136-cfda93.996-cid2319-instructions.doc. Accessed November 17, 2007.

[30] Strategic National Stockpiles (April 14, 2005). Available at: http://www.bt.cdc.gov/stockpile. Accessed March 13, 2007.

[31] Simple Triage and Rapid Treatment (START). Available at: http://www.citmt.org/start/background.htm. Accessed April 11, 2007.

[32] TheJumpSTART Pediatric MCI Triage Tool and other pediatric disaster and emergency medicine resources. Available at: http://www.jumpstarttriage.com. Accessed April 11, 2007.

[33] Romig LE. The JumpSTART Pediatric MCI Triage Tool: principles of multicasualty triage and other pediatric disaster and emergency medicine resources. Team Life Support Inc. Promoting better outcomes for children, families and responders. Available at: http://www.jumpstarttriage.com/JumpSTART_and_MCI_Triage.php. Accessed April 11, 2007.

[34] Columbia University School of Nursing Center for Health Policy. Adapting standards of care under altered conditions. Prepared for the American Nurses Association. Privileged communication for comments only. September 27, 2007. When finalized will be available at: www.nursingworld.com.

[35] Phillips SJ, Knebel A, editors. Mass medical care with scarce resources: a community planning guide. Available at: http://www.ahrq.gov/research/mce/mceguide.pdf. Accessed April 30, 2007.

[36] Basic disaster life support. Available at: http://www.emhelpcenter.org/bdls_information.html. Accessed April 30, 2007.

ELSEVIER
SAUNDERS

Crit Care Nurs Clin N Am 20 (2008) 103–109

CRITICAL CARE
NURSING CLINICS
OF NORTH AMERICA

# Directions for Disaster Nursing Education in the United States

Marguerite T. Littleton-Kearney, PhD, RN, FAAN[a,b,*],
Lynn A. Slepski, MSN, RN, CCNS, USPHS[c]

[a]Department of Acute and Chronic Care, Johns Hopkins School of Nursing, Baltimore, MD, USA
[b]Department of Anesthesia/Critical Care Medicine, Johns Hopkins School of Medicine, Baltimore, MD, USA
[c]U.S. Public Health Service, Risk Management and Analysis Department of Homeland Security, Washington, DC, USA

The potential for a high-impact incident resulting in mass casualties remains a specter plaguing the health care system. The increasing frequency of natural disasters and world-wide terrorist events has emphasized the need for adequate preparation of health care providers in the event that such an incident occurs. Nurses comprise a large percentage of the health care workforce, so that adequate educational preparation for nurses is essential. Yet recent studies [1,2] indicate that nurses remain unprepared to adequately respond to a high-impact event.

Immediately after the attacks on the World Trade Center in New York and the anthrax exposures in the eastern United States, there was an explosion of courses focused on the elements of chemical, biological, radiological, and nuclear terrorism, collectively known as weapons of mass destruction. Emerging infections (eg, severe acute respiratory syndrome [SARS]), the threat of pandemic viral influenza (eg, Avian influenza), and the frequent occurrence of natural disasters, however, have emphasized the fact that these events may result in an influx of the sick or injured equaling or exceeding the number associated with weapons of mass destruction. Consequently, many educational programs for health

care professionals now use the all-hazards approach. Education for nurses, built on the all-hazards approach, provides the framework for college nursing program curricula, and for continuing education (CE) and just-in-time instruction.

## Educational demand

Before 2001, few nurses received any formal education in the areas of emergency preparedness or disaster response. Nurses who did possess some rudimentary knowledge likely served in the military, worked as prehospital providers, were employed in a hospital emergency department, or participated in humanitarian disaster relief work. Consequently, most nurses graduating from schools before 2001 have wide gaps in their knowledge of disaster care.

It is accepted that any event resulting in mass illness or injury will exceed the number of health care workers able to supply care. Nurses comprise the largest number of health care workers, but many nurses are unprepared to respond because of lack of knowledge or skills. These existing deficits create a nursing workforce requiring additional hours of formal instruction to be able to respond effectively in the event of a high-impact incident resulting in mass casualties. It is accepted that all practicing nurses should possess a basic understanding and skill set to be able to provide care in the event of a mass casualty event [3]. These educational demands are staggering, particularly in a health care environment already

* Corresponding author. Johns Hopkins University School of Nursing, 625 North Wolfe Street, Baltimore, MD 21205, USA.

*E-mail address:* mkearne2@son.jhmi.edu (M.T. Littleton-Kearney).

0899-5885/08/$ - see front matter. Published by Elsevier Inc.
doi:10.1016/j.ccell.2007.10.008

operating at or above capacity. Innovative ways to educate nurses and other health professionals are being instituted. At least three national CE courses targeting physicians, dentists, paramedics, and nurses were created and are now offered nationally under the sponsorship of the American Medical Association [4]. Patterned on the basic and advanced life support course model, these courses and have three levels: core disaster life support (CDLS), basic disaster life support (BDLS) and advanced disaster life support (ADLS). These programs, however, may be unavailable in more rural locations. Additionally, they can be costly, and many nurses cannot get paid time off work to attend the courses.

Computer-based training, a strategy used in many fields of study, is another newer alternative for practicing nurses to augment their disaster training. On-line training has been purported to be more efficacious, more convenient and more flexible, because it can be completed at the learner's own time and pace [5]. These electronic resources typically include on-line, learn at one's own pace modules [5], and many are offered free of charge. Upon completion of many of these computer modules, the learner can print a certificate to show proof of training. A basic review of nurses' responsibilities during disasters is sponsored jointly by the American Red Cross and Sigma Theta Tau International, but this on-line course provides very basic information and should be considered a starting point for further more in-depth education (http://www.nursingsociety.org/education/case_studies/cases/SP0004.htmlwww.nursingsociety.org). The Centers for Disease Control and Prevention (CDC) offer excellent information on chemical, biological, and radiological emergencies, and the information can be accessed easily from the CDC Web site. Two nursing groups, the International Nursing Coalition for Mass Casualty Education (INCMCE; as of spring 2007 changed to Nursing Emergency Preparedness Education Coalition, NEPEC) and the National Nurse Emergency Preparedness Initiative (NNEPI), are excellent sources of computer links for many of these Web-based training modules relevant for nurses.

Although numerous computer-based training modules for health professionals exist, most of these on-line educational offerings do not specifically target nurses. With funding from the Agency for Healthcare and Quality (AHRQ), Elizabeth Weiner was one of the first individuals to spearhead the development of six disaster education modules specific for nurses [5]. All the modules were developed and centered on the core competencies for practicing nurses identified by INCMCE/NEPEC. Access to these free modules is obtained at the INCMCE Web site (www.incmce.org). Another recent computer-based initiative specifically for nurses is under construction by NNEPI (www.nnepi.org) and funded by the US Department of Homeland Security. Similar to the INCMCE/NEPEC modules, the NNEPI on-line program consists of six modules taking about 6 hours to complete. These free modules are nearing completion, and it is anticipated that they will be available on-line in the near future. Another innovative CE program of study can be accessed on-line at St. Louis University (http://nursing.slu.edu/cne_disaster_prep_home.html). Completion of this nurse-focused CE program provides a certificate in disaster preparedness. Nurses desiring to obtain a certificate are required to pay a fee and must complete six required and four elective modules (from a list of 12). Many other on-line disaster training programs not specifically targeted to nurses are widely available, and both NEPEC and NNEPI have links to the Web sites.

Although the need to educate nurses in the fundamentals of disaster care is recognized, and great strides have been made, nursing school curriculum in the United States for the most part remains inadequate [6]. Weiner and colleagues [6] showed that as late as 2003, the number of hours focused on the nurse's role in disaster preparedness in American schools of nursing had increased marginally, but continued to be inadequate. They identified several important obstacles for this including: curricula already heavily content laden, lack of scholarly articles targeted for nurses, inadequately defined and validated fundamental content, and faculty insufficiently prepared to teach the content [5]. Nevertheless, some university-based schools of nursing are attempting to integrate disaster nursing content throughout the curriculum, often as part of community health course content, or as electives for students to choose [7–9]. For example, the Long Island University School of Nursing involves senior nursing students in a 3-hour lecture covering basic disaster management principles and a 1-day symposium as part of their community health experience [10]. Another school, the Texas Tech University Health Sciences Center School of Nursing, had nursing students participate in a simulated mass causality drill to allow students an opportunity to practice skills [11]. The question remains, however, how much and what type of content is sufficient? Jennings-Sanders and colleagues [9] suggest that short lectures do not provide enough time to synthesize disaster nursing principles. Consequently, they propose that disaster nursing should be a required semester-long course for undergraduate nursing students. This may be very difficult to achieve, because most undergraduate curricula are content-overloaded.

Efforts to expand and formalize essential disaster-related content have been hampered by the fact that no consensus exists concerning fundamental elements, how the content is taught best, or how to promote retention of an overwhelming amount of information. To date, some anecdotal evidence exists to support the efficacy of bioterrorism and disaster preparedness courses [8,10], but a systematic analysis of relevant curricular threads has yet to be completed. This emphasizes that core content for nursing curriculum needs to continue to be delineated and that outcome competencies must be identified and then validated through research. Creation of such a framework then can guide curriculum organization and design. One of the major impediments in the establishment of such a framework is the fact that essential content for disaster nursing education remains poorly characterized; however, preliminary work on competencies is well underway.

## Competencies

The fundamental content of emergency preparedness curricula remains controversial. When considering emergency preparedness training in the hospital setting for example, Rubin questioned not only the quantity of training, but also the usefulness and realistic nature of existing competencies. Although both the American Nurses Association [12] and the American Association of Colleges of Nursing [13] recommend appropriate basic education and continued education for all nurses in emergency preparedness, neither define content.

So, what is meant by competencies? Core competencies are defined as the knowledge, skills, abilities, and behaviors needed to carry out a job [14]. Articulated by measurable statements, competencies are based on key essential job functions, frequently used job functions and accountabilities, and high-risk job functions and accountabilities that involve actions that could cause harm, death or legal actions to customers, employees, or the organization. Whitcomb [15] emphasized that core competencies delineate the knowledge, skills, and attitudes that learners must acquire to be able

to perform within each competency domain at a predetermined level. Attaining competencies helps to ensure that programs achieve certain outcomes.

Several authors suggest the development of formal emergency preparedness educational core competencies [16–18] with competency-based objective evaluation [19]. A second group suggests that emergency preparedness training should be required CE [20–22] or a requisite for medical privileges or licensure [23]. The Joint Commission on the Accreditation of Healthcare Organizations (JCAHO) requires measurement of competency in its accreditation process [24]. In January 2001, JCAHO introduced new emergency management standards, building on its long-standing disaster preparedness requirements [24]. One specific phase of the new standard includes determination of the priorities for, and means for effectively deploying, the finite resources needed to support response systems, including trained personnel.

In the absence of standardized federal criteria, several groups have attempted independently to develop core competencies for various responder types without any attempts to harmonize them. Those addressing health care include emergency medical technicians, emergency physicians and emergency nurses [25], emergency response clinicians [26], hospital workers [27], and public health workers [27]. Those specifically addressing nursing include the Columbia School of Nursing [27] (public health and hospital nurses), the Association of Teachers of Preventive Medicine (2003), (clinicians–nurses and physicians) [26], and INCMCE/NEPEC (general nurses) [28]. Unfortunately, the vision and resulting competency requirements are inconsistent across the groups. Further, no attempt has been made to validate if these competencies are accurate or address the full spectrum of required skill sets—information that is essential for planning and future training.

According to the White House-commissioned Katrina Report [29], the required knowledge, skills, and abilities of health care professionals differed from existing competency lists. The White House report stated:

> "Immediate public health and medical support challenges included the identification, triage, and treatment of acutely sick and injured patients; the management of chronic medical conditions in large number of evacuees with special health care needs; the assessment, communication and mitigation of public health risks; mortuary support;

and the provision of assistance to state and local health officials to quickly reestablish health care deliver systems and public health infrastructures."

Recently the National Organization of Nurse Practitioner Faculties recognized that curricula development for advanced practice nurses (APN) is difficult, as most educators are unfamiliar with emergency preparedness content [30,31], and curricula are already full. As a result, the group has taken a different approach, identifying key emergency preparedness content that can be incorporated into existing courses and providing resources to assist faculty in delivering the content. The white paper should be published soon and will be widely available.

### Educational content

Because disasters are intrinsically unpredictable, complete preparedness for disasters, particularly in the case of a bioterrorism event, is likely not fully attainable [32]. Consequently, the dynamic nature of preparedness makes precise identification of basic educational priorities specific for nurses difficult at best. Nevertheless, since 2001, progress has been made. Existing literature reflects five general elements important for nurses, and several authors suggest that these should be incorporated into curricula [8,33,34]. These educational priorities include: detection and reporting of unusual outbreaks, treatment of ill and injured, control measure implementation, resources and preparedness planning, and management of the public. Interestingly, a landmark study of Wisconsin nurses identified at least eight similar educational priorities for nurses dealing with disasters and other large health care emergencies [1]. Unsurprisingly, the top three priorities dealt with nurses' knowledge of: 1) triage and first aid, 2) detection of symptoms associated with biological agent-caused diseases, and 3) accessing critical resources such as the strategic national stockpile. Other areas where nurses felt undereducated were the incident command system, quarantine, decontamination, psychological first aid, epidemiology, clinical decision-making, and communications/connectivity [1].

To date, three models for disaster nursing have been described. The Jennings-Saunders disaster management model highlights four phases that nurses in the community may use to plan disaster nursing care [35]. Each phase focuses on different aspects of disaster planning and response. While the phase 1 (predisaster) targets planning for disaster and resource allocation, phase 2 (disaster) addresses nurses' role in the midst of a disaster. Phases 3 and 4 of the model deal with health need evaluation and effects of the disaster on patient or population health, respectively [35]. In Veenema's early ground-breaking text, the author uses the typical disaster model phases of preimpact, impact, and postimpact to describe model nursing roles specific for each phase of the disaster [36]. Most recently, Wynd proposed a model for disaster military nursing [37], incorporating elements of both the Jennings and the Veenema models [35,36]. Wynd's model, like Veenema's, focuses on military nursing activities involving preparedness and readiness (phase 1); on impact/response and implementation (phase 2); and finally on postimpact recovery, reconstruction, and re-evaluation (phase 3).

These examples illustrate the progress thus far that nurses and nurse educators have made in the identification of components of core knowledge and practice models necessary for optimal function in the event of large-scale health emergencies. Ground-breaking work already had been accomplished, as evidenced by the publication of the core competencies for public health workers and by INCMCE/NEPEC [3,38]. The next steps will be to design a suggested curriculum for university and continuing education that is widely available and endorsed by all the major nursing accreditation bodies as requisite knowledge for nurses responding to emergencies caused by natural disasters, infectious illness, or terrorism.

### New directions in disaster nursing

Effective response to disasters and other large-scale health emergency requires strong leadership, strategic planning, and interprofessional collaboration. Several schools of nursing recognize the need for graduate education and to that end have created masters degree programs and post-masters certificates in emergency planning and disaster response [39]. The University of Rochester (New York) was the first school of nursing to create a masters program to educate nurses as leaders in disaster response and emergency preparedness [39]. The program focuses on the development of skills leaders need to design, implement, and evaluate programs dealing with emergency response and disaster management. Another trendsetter was the Johns Hopkins

Table 1
Masters degree nursing programs focused on disaster preparedness/disaster response in the United States (in alphabetical order)

| University | Program title | Credits for degree completion |
|---|---|---|
| Adelphi University School of Nursing, Garden City, N.Y. | Emergency Nursing and Disaster Management | 39 credits[a] |
| Columbia University School of Nursing, New York | Emergency Preparedness Response | 45–49 credits masters plus nine credits as emergency preparedness subspecialty |
| Johns Hopkins University School of Nursing, Baltimore, | Health Systems Management: Emergency Preparedness/Disaster Response | 39 credits[a] |
| University of Pittsburgh School of Nursing, Pittsburgh | ACNP: Trauma and Emergency Preparedness | 44–46 credits for ACNP including subspecialty disaster preparedness courses |
| University of Rochester School of Nursing, Rochester, N.Y. | Leadership in Health Care Systems in Disaster Response and Emergency Preparedness | 30 credits |
| University of Tennessee College of Nursing, Knoxville, Tenn. | Homeland Security Nursing | 37 credits (CNS)[a] <br> 56 credits (NP)[a] |
| Vanderbilt University School of Nursing, Nashville, Tenn. | Health Systems Management | 39 credits, plus six credits elective concentration |

*Abbreviations:* ACNP, acute care nurse practitioner; CNS, clinical nurse specialist.
[a] Post-masters certificate option.

School of Nursing (JHUSON, Baltimore), which in fall 2005 inaugurated what is believed to be the first nursing graduate program geared toward the preparation of nurse leaders in emergency response and disaster management in health care facilities. The masters track was established on the belief that nurses always have held key positions in health care facilities, that they possess valuable insider knowledge of how health care facilities function during disasters, and that they hold pivotal roles in the formulation of institutional disaster management plans. Students are required to complete courses on health systems management, education, national/international humanitarian relief, emergency planning, and disaster response (a series of three). A 12 credit post-masters certificate is also available. Concurrent to the initiation of the JHUSON masters program, the University of Tennessee at Knoxville also launched a nursing masters degree and post-masters certificate option in homeland security nursing. Students may opt to focus their studies on management or on advanced practice/ clinical nurse specialist roles. The post-masters option requires completion of 24 credits. Adelphi University (Garden City, Long Island, N. Y.) recently started a masters/post-masters degree in emergency nursing and disaster management.

Other university schools of nursing offer masters track subspecialty options or post-masters certificates, including Columbia University and University of Pittsburg (Table 1). As more university schools of nursing expand their masters options to include specialty tracks in emergency response and disaster preparedness, it is likely that graduates will assume groundbreaking new roles as health care leaders, emergency planners, biopreparedness coordinators, and educators.

## Summary

Educating nurses to meet the challenge of dealing with patients from large-scale health emergencies such as natural disasters, infectious disease outbreaks, and chemical, biological, and radiological terrorism always will be difficult based on the unpredictable nature of such events. Content development is complicated further, because few researched-based studies validating the efficacy and retention of emergency preparedness training/education are published. Consequently, much of the work in this area is accessible only through preliminary (and often unpublished) reports at conferences and therefore unavailable for use by nursing faculty, policy makers, decision makers, and researchers.

Fundamental to a comprehensive and effective national training plan for nurses and other health care professionals is consensus about the operational definitions of emergency preparedness. Heightened understanding of all the components of emergency preparedness education ensures that the range of preincident actions and processes are: standardized and consistent with mutually agreed upon doctrine and measurable, resulting in integrated emergency preparedness education. Additionally, there should be training exercises incorporating nationally formulated core competencies across all responder/receiver roles. Once this preliminary work is completed, more attention needs to be devoted to rigorous scientific evaluation of the effectiveness of existing emergency preparedness education programs. In addition, systems of metrics to detail capacity and performance must be created. These have significant implications for the future development of educational programs in this area. Although it is virtually impossible to completely prepare every nurse to respond to all types of large-scale health crises, it is possible to identify comprehensive emergency preparedness principles that can provide a framework for university curriculum, CE programs, and just-in-time training, thus creating a nursing workforce better equipped to respond when disasters do strike.

# References

[1] Wisniewski R, Dennik-Champion G, Peltier JW. Emergency preparedness competencies. J Nurs Adm 2004;54(10):475–80.

[2] Katz AR, Nekorchuk DM, Holck PS, et al. Hawaii physician and nurse bioterrorism preparedness survey. Prehospital Disaster Med 2006;21(6):404–13.

[3] Stanley J. Disaster competency development and integration in nursing education. Nurs Clin North Am 2005;40:453–67.

[4] Colvard MD, Naiman MI, Mara D, et al. Disaster medicine training survey results for dental health care providers in Illinois. J Am Dent Assoc 2007; 138(4):519–24.

[5] Weiner E. Preparing nurses internationally for emergency planning and response. Online J Issues Nurs 2006;11(3) Available at: www.nursingworld.org. ojin/topic31/tpc31_3.htm.

[6] Weiner E, Irwin M, Trangenstein P, et al. Emergency preparedness curriculum in nursing schools in the United States. Nurs Educ Perspect 2005; 26(6):332–9.

[7] Pattillo MM. Mass casualty disaster nursing course. Nurse Educ 2003;28(6):271–5.

[8] Steed CJ, Howe LA, Pruitt RH, et al. Integrating bioterrorism education into nursing school curricula. J Nurs Educ 2004;43(3):362–7.

[9] Jennings-Sanders A, Frisch N, Wing S. Nursing students' perceptions about disaster nursing. Disaster Manag Response 2005;3(3):80–5.

[10] Ireland M, Emerson EA, Kontzamanis E, et al. Integrating disaster preparedness into a community health nursing course: one school's experience. Disaster Manag Response 2006;4(3):72–6.

[11] Decker SI, Galvan TJ, Sridaromont K. Integrating an exercise on mass casualty response into the curriculum. J Nurs Educ 2005;44(7):339–40.

[12] American Nurses Association. Action report: the nursing profession and disaster preparedness. Presented at the American Nurses Association 2002 House of Delegates meeting. Philadelphia, June 28–July 1, 2002. Available at: http://www.nursingworld. orgabout/hod02/actions.htm. Accessed June 22, 2004.

[13] American Association of Colleges of Nursing. American Association of Colleges of Nursing Leads Efforts to Further the Education of Nurses to Combat Bioterrorism (2001, November 1). Available at: http://www.aacn.nche.edu/Media/NewsReleases/ bioterrorism.htm. Accessed June 22, 2004.

[14] Wright D. The ultimate guide to competency assessment in healthcare. 2nd edition. Minneapolis (MN): Creative Healthcare Management; 1998.

[15] Whitcomb ME. More on competency-based education. Acad Med 2004;79(6):493–4.

[16] Chafee M, Conway-Welch C, Sabatier K. Nursing leaders plan to educate nurses about response to mass casualty events. Am Nurse 2001; Available at: http://www.nursingworld.org/tan/01julaug/casualty. htm. Accessed June 22, 2004.

[17] Gebbie KM, Qureshi K. Emergency and disaster preparedness: core competencies for nurses. Am J Nurs 2002;102(1):46–51.

[18] Tilson H, Gebbie KM. The public health workforce. Annu Rev Public Health 2004;25:241–56.

[19] Trautman D, Watson JE. Implementing continued clinical competency evaluation in the emergency department. J Nurs Staff Dev 1995;11(1):41–7.

[20] Croasdale M. Doctor interest in bioterrorism is wearing off. Am Med News 2002;45(24):9–10.

[21] Hilton C, Allison V. Disaster preparedness: an indictment for action by nursing educators. J Contin Educ Nurs 2004;35(2) 59-5.

[22] Jones J, Terndrup TE, Franz DR, et al. Future challenges in preparing for and responding to bioterrorism events. Emerg Med Clin North Am 2002;20(2): 501–24.

[23] Shadel BN, Clements B, Arndt B, et al. What we need to know about bioterrorism preparedness: results from focus groups conducted at APIC 2000. Am J Infect Control 2001;29(6):347–51.

[24] Joint Commission on the Accreditation of Healthcare Organizations. Mobilizing America's health care reservoir. Jt Comm Perspect 2001;21(12).

Available at: http://www.jcrinc.com/subscribers/ perspectives.asp?durki=2512&site=10&return=1122. Accessed June 22, 2004.

[25] NBC Task Force. Final report: developing objectives, content and competencies for the training of emergency medical technicians, emergency physicians, and emergency nurses to care for casualties resulting from nuclear, biological, or chemical (NBC) incidents. Washington, DC: Government Printing Office; 2001.

[26] Association of Teachers of Preventive Medicine (2003, July). Emergency response clinician. Available at: http://www.atpm.org/education/ Clinical_Compt.html. Accessed June, 2007.

[27] Columbia School of Nursing. Emergency preparedness competencies (annotated); Public Health Professionals. New York: Center for Health Policy; 2001. p. 745–750.

[28] Stanley JM. Directions for nursing education. In: Veenema TG, editor. Disaster nursing and emergency preparedness for chemical, biological, and radiological terrorism and other hazards. New York: Springer; 2003. p. 461–71.

[29] Townsend FF. The federal response to Hurricane Katrina: lessons learned. 2006; Available at: http:// www.whitehouse.gov/reports/katrina-lessons-learned/. Accessed February 28, 2006.

[30] Rubin JN. Recurring pitfalls in hospital preparedness and response. J Homeland Security 2004; Available at: http://www.homelandsecurity.org/newjournal/ articles/rubin.html Accessed January 13, 2004.

[31] Veenema TG. Chemical and biological terrorism preparedness for staff development specialists. J Nurs Staff Dev 2002;19(5):215–22.

[32] Rebmann T. Defining bioterrorism preparedness for nurses: concept analysis. J Adv Nurs 2006;54(5): 623–32.

[33] O'Connell KP, Menuey BC, Foster D. Issues in preparedness for biological terrorism. A perspective for critical care nursing. AACN Clin Issues 2002;13: 425–69.

[34] Rose MA, Larrimore KL. Knowledge and awareness concerning chemical and biological terrorism: continuing education implications. J Contin Educ Nurs 2002;33:253–8.

[35] Jennings-Saunders A. Teaching disaster nursing by utilizing the Jennings disaster management model. Nurs Educ Pract 2003;4 69-6.

[36] Veenema TG. Disaster nursing and emergency preparedness fro chemical, biological and radiological terrorism and other hazards. New York: Springer Publishing; 2003. p. 9.

[37] Wynd CA. A proposed model for military disaster nursing. Online J Issues Nurs 2006;11(3). Available at: www.nursingworld.org.ojin/topic31/tpc31_4. htm.

[38] Gebbie K, Merrill J. Public health worker competencies for emergency response. J Pub Health Adm 2002;8(3) 73–1.

[39] Veenema TG. Expanding educational opportunities in disaster responses and emergency preparedness for nurses. Nurs Educ Perspect 2006;27(2):93–9.

ELSEVIER
SAUNDERS

Crit Care Nurs Clin N Am 20 (2008) 111–119

CRITICAL CARE
NURSING CLINICS
OF NORTH AMERICA

# Research Considerations When Studying Disasters

Catherine Wilson Cox, RN, PhD, CCRN, CEN, CCNS,
CAPT, NC, USN (RC)

*School of Nursing & Health Studies, Georgetown University, 3700 Reservoir Road NW, Washington, DC 20057, USA*

Nurses play an integral role during disasters because they, more than any other health care professional, are called upon during disaster response efforts. Consequently, nurse researchers are interested in studying the issues that impact nurses in the aftermath of a disaster [1,2]. "Disaster nursing requires new concepts of what constitutes good care" [2]. For example, in a disaster situation, care shifts from concentrating resuscitative efforts on the sickest patients to conserving one's resources and caring for the majority of the victims. Disaster nurses know when to make this shift, and nurse researchers are challenged to define additional concepts that exemplify disaster nursing [2]. Thus, this article offers research considerations for nurse scientists when developing proposals related to disaster research and identifies resources and possible sources of funding for their projects.

## Disaster research methods

The majority of disaster studies have been descriptive [1], because "conducting methodologically rigorous studies of responses to disasters and other traumatic life events is extraordinarily challenging" [3]. The challenges of disaster research include obtaining external funding, especially for quick-response grants; gaining access to traumatized patients; the unpredictability of these events; and working with institutional review boards

(IRBs) [3]. Hence, one set of researchers proposes an Internet-based approach to community epidemiologic studies as a partial solution to these challenges [3]. These investigators call for a rapid research response after disasters and note that telephone and Internet surveys can be implemented quickly and are more efficient than traditional in-person survey interview methods. This method allows findings to be published more quickly, as was the case when four papers using these methods and describing reactions to the events of September 11, 2001 appeared in top-tiered journals within a year. By contrast, papers related to the Oklahoma City bombing in 1995, which were based on in-person interviews, did not appear in the literature until 1999. The authors' original article provides more information on how the Internet can enhance disaster study design [3].

There is no doubt that a disaster research study that includes probability sampling increases external validity (or generalizability of the findings) [3]. The challenge in drawing probability samples is that the two most popular methods—home address and random-digit dialing—require that, after the disaster, a study participant have a house to come back to and/or a land-line telephone. The Internet has its own inherent problems, in that only 60% of the population in the United States has access to it; therefore, a group surveyed using the Internet does not represent the United States population [3]. Moreover, any loss of power after a disaster would make data collection over the Internet impossible.

Incidentally, a meta-analysis of 225 disaster studies found the following sampling strategies: 31% convenience, 6% clinical, 17% purposive, 19% probability, and 27% census [4]. Less than

The views expressed in this article are those of the author and do not reflect the official policy of the Department of the Navy, the Department of Defense, or the United States Government.

*E-mail address:* cathicox@aol.com

0899-5885/08/$ - see front matter. Published by Elsevier Inc.
doi:10.1016/j.ccell.2007.10.003

one third of the samples were assessed more than once after the disaster, and only a few were assessed before the disaster. The literature was replete with short- and intermediate-term disaster effects, but there were few data on the long-term effects. Finally, the meta-analysis revealed small sample sizes (median sample size, 150); thus, these studies lacked power [4]. Certainly, disaster research needs more studies with longitudinal designs that allow assessments to be compared before exposure and provide multiple postexposure contacts [3].

### The privacy rule

The Health Insurance Portability and Accountability Act (HIPAA) of 1996, which was implemented in 2003, mandates the protection of identifiable health information for patients and includes a federal regulation known as the "Privacy Rule." The Website for the Department of Health and Human Services' Office for Civil Rights' [5] provides up-to-date information on the Privacy Rule, including a decision-making tool to help the researcher understand whether the rule should be applied, based on whether the research is associated with a "covered entity" [6]. Covered entities include hospitals, health plans, and health care workers who electronically transmit protected health information (PHI) [1]. Because most nurses work for or are associated with a covered entity, they need to adhere to the Privacy Rule [1].

The application of the Privacy Rule depends on the setting and the data collected. If the study involves PHI, the Privacy Rule applies. If, however, the study looks at nursing functions, without the use of PHI, the Privacy Rule does not apply. Additionally, because surveys and interviews generally do not result in the creation of PHI, they are not subjected to the Privacy Rule [1].

The Privacy Rule could impede new knowledge because it would require obtaining authorization from each individual involved in the study before that PHI could be used; however, covered entities usually are not required to obtain written authorization if the PHI is used for research, as long as an IRB approves a waiver and the researcher details how the PHI will be handled. Most disaster research studies are not affected by the HIPAA Privacy Rule, given the nature of disaster research, as long as these studies receive waivers [1].

### Protection of human subjects from research risk

Federal regulations mandate that research involving human subjects address the risk to participants, the adequacy of protection against these risks, the potential benefits to the study's participants and others, and the importance of the knowledge gained [6]. These points were discussed in January 2003 when the New York Academy of Medicine and the National Institute of Mental Health (NIMH) sponsored a meeting entitled "Ethical Issues Pertaining to Research in the Aftermath of Disaster." The attendees included "mental health professionals, trauma researchers, public health officials, ethicists, [IRB] representatives, as well as family members and first responders from the Oklahoma City and World Trade Center disasters" [7]. The panel was tasked with providing recommendations to assist researchers in conducting postdisaster research in a safe and ethical manner [7].

The benefits and risks associated with participation in postdisaster research that the symposium attendees considered are listed in Box 1. "[S]ince research [post-disaster] is not always intended to benefit present participants researchers must remember that subjects bear the burdens and risks of research in order to benefit future persons who will experience a disaster" [7].

Regarding the possibility of emotional distress, one set of investigators point out that most participants in trauma-related studies do not experience strong negative emotions when studied; however, the experience of previous distress, being relatively young or old, having a history of more than one trauma exposure, or having suffered severe physical injury may predispose responders to experiencing emotional distress when participating in research related to traumatic events [8]. Researchers need to be mindful of the timing of their inquires, waiting for survivors to bury their dead, obtain housing if lost during the event, confer with relief agencies, and/or report their losses to their insurance companies [9].

Any investigator considering postdisaster research should consult the article by Collogan and colleagues [7] for 12 points recommended by the attendees of the symposium. One of the most important points is that, as a group, those affected by a disaster have decision-making capacity to consent voluntarily to the research. This aspect is confirmed in the literature [10]. Another important point is that disaster-affected populations should not be automatically considered

---

**Box 1. Benefits and risks of participating in postdisaster research**

*Benefits*
Enhanced awareness of material resources
Medical and mental health services
Empowerment
Learning and insight
Altruism
Kinship with others
Feeling of satisfaction or value after participating
Favorable attention from investigators

*Risks*
Physical harm
Inconvenience
Legal action
Economic hardship
Psychologic discomfort
Loss of dignity
Breach of confidentiality
Unwanted media attention
Overburden to individuals caused by multiple or repetitive studies
Emotional distress
Pressure to consent to research to avoid appearing unpatriotic or unhelpful

---

*Data from* Collogan LK, Tuma F, Dolan-Sewell R, et al. Ethical issues pertaining to research in the aftermath of disaster. Journal of Traumatic Stress 2004;17(5):363–72.

---

"vulnerable," as defined in federal regulations; however, the research staff should be trained to recognize when mental health consultation is warranted, a concept that also is clarified in the literature [11]. Kilpatrick [12] summarizes this issue:

> It is incumbent upon all of us to base our decisions about research and protection of research participants on facts—not opinions. Our opinions may tell us that this type of research is inherently risky, but the facts say otherwise. Risks to participants are generally not great, and these risks can be managed by thoughtful researchers.

Researchers should keep in mind that racial and ethnic populations in the United States may be more vulnerable to natural disasters by virtue of "language, housing patterns, building construction, community isolation, and cultural insensitivities" [13].

IRBs may find themselves in a tough position when evaluating disaster research protocols. They must evaluate the soundness of proposals and also must balance federal regulations with the desire of the principal investigator (PI) to start data collection as soon as possible. If data collection is to occur at multiple sites, researchers will need to allot more time for multiple IRB reviews [1], possibly forfeiting the chance to begin data collection immediately. In reality, it would be virtually impossible for a PI to obtain IRB approval for a proposal immediately after a disaster. Thus, one of the best strategies would be to develop a proposal based on the researcher's area of interest and have it preapproved before the actual event. This process is similar to the mechanism used by the University of Colorado, Boulder when evaluating quick-response grant proposals [14].

**Resources**

*Natural hazards center*

The National Science Foundation sponsors the Quick Response Program. This funding opportunity is designed to provide travel, per diem, and modest data collection costs for social and behavioral scientists in the United States who want to go to a disaster site quickly to collect data. These small grants (which average $2000.00) are available only to study disasters as they are happening or during the immediate aftermath (eg, within weeks of impact). The Natural Hazards Center at the University of Colorado, Boulder administers this program, and it requires that proposals (limited to three pages) be submitted and preapproved before a disaster. Because one cannot easily anticipate a disaster, the Center encourages researchers to identify a topic area (eg, response and recovery times) that can be studied no matter where the disaster occurs or what type it is. This strategy makes the proposal more likely to be preapproved and eventually implemented but requires the researcher to anticipate disasters on an annual basis. If the disaster occurs within the allotted time period, the researcher contacts the Center for authorization to go to the field. If the disaster does not occur during the calendar year of the program, the proposal must be reviewed and revised, including updating the PI's curriculum vitae, assuming the PI wants to resubmit the application [14].

*Advancing disaster research*

In June 2004, the Disaster Research Education Mentoring (DREM) Center was established, funded by the NIMH and the National Institute for Nursing Research. It is one of three projects developed for enhancing disaster research. Its primary function is to provide technical assistance as well as educate and mentor researchers studying disasters and terrorism. The DREM Center boasts experienced scientists who have solid disaster research records, and its Website offers detailed information regarding three steps to take when designing and conducting a research project after a disaster and/or a terrorist attack (Box 2) [15].

The second project designed to enhance disaster research is Research Education in Disaster Mental Health, funded in 2003 by the NIMH. Its goals are

> to inform, instruct, advise, and mentor disaster researchers. On [its Website researchers] will find research summaries to inform the scientific community about topics salient after major disasters, instructional materials such as summaries from a book on research education in disaster mental health, contact information for those looking for advising on a particular project, and information

about a mentoring program for promising newcomers to the field [16].

The third project designed to enhance disaster research is the Disaster Research Training grant.

> The goal of this program is to enhance the nation's capacity for conducting rapid post-event disaster mental health research related to children and families through training of researchers and responder organizations in state-of the-art research methods, emphasizing methods of needs assessment, data collection, clinical evaluation, surveillance treatment and intervention, and evaluations of effectiveness [16].

The Disaster Research Training program is linked to the National Child Traumatic Stress Network, which collaborates with academic and community-based service centers to develop and disseminate evidenced-based interventions [17].

*National Institutes of Health funding opportunity announcement*

A 2006 funding opportunity announcement was released on behalf of three organizations within the National Institutes of Health: the National Institute on Aging, the National Institute for Nursing Research, and National Institute of Child Health and Human Development. It calls for proposals to study the consequences of natural and manmade disasters regarding the health of vulnerable populations, including children and the elderly. Table 1 offers suggested research topics. If a PI requires a quick response when answering a National Institutes of Health notice following a disaster, the application may be expedited; however, the submission of letters of intent and sponsorship agreements are required [6].

**Fieldwork**

Collecting data after a disaster may require fieldwork, including ethnography. With ethnography, the researcher is immersed in a setting for a period of time to understand the phenomenon of interest [18]. Ethnography's roots come from anthropology; anthropologists periodically lived with the natives to understand their point of view. Today, participant observation can range from detached and impersonal to interactive and participative [19]. Controversy exists as to whether nurse researchers should participate in the experience rather than simply documenting and reflecting on it [18,19]. This dilemma

---

**Box 2. The Disaster Research Education Mentoring Center's three steps to take in preparation for a research project**

*Steps*

1. Collect up-to-date information on the disaster. Relevant questions include:
   What happened?
   Where did the disaster take place?
   What populations seem to be most affected?
   How many people died from the disaster?
   How many people were injured in the disaster?
   How many people have been displaced?
   How much property damage did the disaster cause?
   Was there a warning of the disaster?
   What rescue efforts have been established?
   Are many people seeking services?
   What is the state response?
   Is there an international response? What is it?
Resources include background Websites:
http://firstgov.gov
http://redcross.org
http://disasterhelp.gov
http://www.bt.cdc.gov/index.asp
http://www.hhs.gov/disasters
2. Become familiar with the literature surrounding postdisaster research.
   The Disaster Research Education Mentoring Center offers free postdisaster research
      publications, but one needs to contact the Center for passwords to access the articles.
3. Explore funding options and create partnerships in research projects. Potential funding
   sources include:
   The Annie E. Casey Foundation
   The Center for Health Care Strategies
   The Centers for Disease Control
   The Commonwealth Fund
   The Ford Foundation
   The Foundation Center
   The International Research & Exchanges Board
   The National Institutes of Health
   The National Institute of Nursing Research
   The National Institute on Drug Abuse
   The Rockefeller Foundation
   The Robert Wood Johnson Foundation
   The Substance Abuse & Mental Health Services Administration
   The US Department of Health and Human Services GrantsNet
   The WK Kellogg Foundation

---

   *Data from* Disaster Research Education and Mentoring (DREM) Center. Available at: http://www.
disasterresearch.org. Accessed August 18, 2007.

---

requires nurse researchers to anticipate whether participation in the experience involves a risk for losing data during its collection (eg, being asked to assist with nursing tasks while recording events) and to balance that risk against the study participants' trust and acceptance gained when the researcher demonstrates competency as a nurse.

Table 1
Data from the 2006 Funding opportunity announcement from National Institutes of Health

| Agency | Mission and/or research interests | Suggested (but not limited to) topics |
|---|---|---|
| National Institute on Aging | To improve health and well being of older Americans through research | Not specifically listed in the funding opportunity announcement |
| National Institute for Nursing Research | Encompasses an interest in research that will improve the quality of life and health outcomes for all persons affected by events such as natural disasters, environmental hazards, and other emergency situations | Models and interventions to improve the quality of life and function of persons affected by events such as natural disasters, environmental hazards, and other emergency situations |
| | | Interventions to enhance preparedness and self-management in persons who have disability and chronic illness in disaster situations |
| | | Interventions to assist caregivers of ill and disabled persons to prepare for and respond to disaster situations |
| | | Interventions for acutely ill individuals during and after a disaster |
| | | Management of symptoms in the immediate aftermath of a disaster and postdisaster |
| National Institute of Child Health and Human Development | To ensure that all children have the chance to achieve their full potential for healthy and productive lives, free from disease or disability, and to ensure the health, productivity, independence, and well being of all people through optimum rehabilitation | The effects of demographic characteristics on responses to disasters, including the role of migration, population distribution and density, and the effects of disasters on demographic characteristics |
| | | The role of family and community in mediating and moderating the effects of disasters on children and other vulnerable populations |
| | | Strategies for ensuring the continued health and well being of vulnerable populations including children, homeless and incarcerated populations, non–English-speaking populations, and children and adults who have disabilities and chronic diseases, during and after disasters |
| | | The development and evaluation of culturally relevant, developmentally appropriate intervention methodologies used in postdisaster settings, including educational materials and the role of the media in preserving children's emotional well being |
| | | Investigation of risk and resilience factors associated with children's physical, mental, and behavioral responses to disasters, including fear, stress, depression, grief, separation anxiety, and posttraumatic stress reaction |
| | | The dissemination of pediatric postdisaster research findings and translation into rapid response efforts |

| Other National Institutes of Health research interests | Effects of disaster on vulnerable populations (eg, the homeless, incarcerated populations, non–English-speaking populations, acutely ill persons in hospitals or other institutional settings, and children and adults who have disabilities and chronic diseases) |
| --- | --- |
| | Characteristics of public health systems, acute care, rehabilitation, and long-term care institutions affecting survival, successful evacuation or referral, and continuity of care for the frail elderly, disabled, or chronically ill persons |
| | The impact of neighborhood, household, and family characteristics, including social cohesion and social networks, on survival, successful evacuation, and resettlement or relocation of the elderly, children, the disabled, and the chronically ill; disruption and adaptation of caregiver relationships |
| | Social, economic, and racial/ethnic disparities affecting access to vaccines and other preventive services or affecting the survival, evacuation, resettlement, or relocation of the elderly, children, the disabled, and chronically ill persons |
| | The economic impact on health of disasters, using existing studies with high-quality predisaster assessments of income and assets |
| | Cognitive and other factors affecting risk perceptions and communication, preparedness, and evacuation, relocation, and resettlement decisions |
| | Long-term health impacts of stressful events and factors affecting resiliency and recovery |
| | Simulations and models of disasters and response, elucidating impacts on the elderly and children |
| | Creation of data resources, including self-report data from affected families and persons, emergency responders, health and long-term care providers, and administrative data from medical and other organizations, to improve the infrastructure for behavioral, social, and services research on the health impacts of disasters |

*From* United States Department of Health and Human Services, National Institutes of Health. Behavioral and social research on disasters and health funding opportunity announcement. Available at: http://grants.nih.gov/grants/guide/pa-files/PA-06–452.html. Accessed August 1, 2007.

---

**Box 3. Safety guidelines for field researchers from the University of California, Berkeley**

*General field safety guidelines*
1. Prepare a written plan before you leave, which should include:
   - Your activities
   - Your itinerary
   - Contact information (eg, telephone number, e-mail address, and physical address):
     - At the field site
     - For a primary person at your institution should anything happen
     - For a significant other should anything happen
2. Assemble safety provisions for trip:
   - First aid kit and first aid manual
   - Medications
   - Allergy treatments (if you have allergies)
   - Sunscreen and hat
   - Water purification tablets or filter devices
   - Bug spray
   - Vehicle emergency kit
   - Flashlight
   - Flares
   - Two-way radio (if you will be working alone in an isolated or dangerous area)
   - Personal protective equipment for fieldwork activities (eg, safety glasses/goggles, gloves, hard hat, sturdy work boots)
3. Verify travel immunizations
4. Clarify health insurance coverage and anticipate where to go should an injury occur
5. Obtain travel insurance
6. When outside of the United States, register with the local police station and/or embassy
7. Always carry a photo identification card

*Physical and environmental hazards*
Please refer to original source for the prevention and treatment of dehydration, impure water, sunburn, heat exhaustion, heat stroke, frostbite, hypothermia, carbon monoxide, high-altitude sickness, poisonous plants, military conflict in a foreign country, robbery, theft, and/or assault.

*Animals and pests, including snakes*
1. Keep garbage in rodent-proof containers and stored away from the campsite or work area.
2. Food crumbs and debris may attract insects and animals.
3. Thoroughly shake all clothing and bedding before use.
4. Do not camp or sleep near obvious animal nests or burrows.
5. Carefully look for pests before placing hands, feet, or body in areas where pests live or hide (eg, woodpiles or crevices).
6. Avoid contact with sick or dead animals.
7. Wear clothes made of tightly woven materials and tuck pants into boots.
8. Wear insect repellent.
9. Minimize use of lights after dark in camp or at the work site because lights may attract pests and animals.
10. Use netting to keep pests away from food and people.
11. Carry a first aid manual and kit on any excursion so bites or stings can be treated.
12. If the pest is poisonous or if the bite does not seem to heal properly, seek medical attention immediately.

*Diseases (eg, viruses, bacteria, fungi, and parasites, including food-borne and vector-borne diseases)*
Please refer to original source for the prevention and treatment of specific diseases. Always check with your health care provider before traveling out of the country to learn about specific health risks for the region in which you will conduct your research.

---

*Data from* Office of Environment, Health & Safety, University of California, Berkeley. Safety guidelines for field researchers. Available at: http://www.ehs.berkeley.edu/pubs/fieldresearchsfty.pdf. Accessed August 18, 2007.

## Safety in the field

For nurse researchers who deploy to the field (eg, the actual disaster site), safety concerns must be addressed, set in place, and followed. The University of California, Berkeley has safety guidelines for field researchers who deploy in North America and also worldwide. These safety guidelines, available on the Internet, consist of four areas of concern, summarized in Box 3 [20]. Additionally, the PI should be notified of any task that seems to be unsafe. If a field worker fears injury or suspects that his/her safety is at risk, the field worker should suspend the task and seek refuge [21].

## Summary

The opportunity for nurse scientists to enter the disaster research field has arrived, especially in this age of natural and manmade disasters, including acts of terrorism. Funding opportunities to study various aspects of disasters do exist; however, writing a research proposal and getting IRB approval immediately after a disaster is an organizational challenge. Thus, nurse researchers should seek preapproval of their studies by anticipating potential disasters and basing their research questions on their area of expertise, instead of focusing on the actual disaster scenario. Additionally, nurse researchers will be best served if they utilize existing resources (eg, the DREM Center and the Research Education in Disaster Mental Health Program) when developing their proposals. Researchers should keep in mind that funding agencies may provide a call for proposals immediately after an event. Finally, nurses can best define nursing practice in the disaster setting by studying it, being mindful to exercise safety in the field.

## References

[1] Lavin RP. HIPAA and disaster research: preparing to conduct research. Disaster Manag Response 2006;4(2):32–7.

[2] NeSmith EG. Defining "disasters" with implications for nursing scholarship and practice. Disaster Manag Response 2006;4(2):59–63.

[3] Schlenger WE, Silver RC. Web-based methods in terrorism and disaster research. J Trauma Stress 2006;19(2):185–93.

[4] Norris FH. Disaster research methods: past progress and future directions. J Trauma Stress 2006;19(2): 173–84.

[5] Office for Civil Rights. Available at: http://www.hhs.gov/OCR. Accessed August 1, 2007.

[6] Behavioral and social research on disasters and health funding opportunity announcement. Available at: http://grants.nih.gov/grants/guide/pa-files/PA-06–452.html. Accessed August 1, 2007.

[7] Collogan LK, Tuma F, Dolan-Sewell R, et al. Ethical issues pertaining to research in the aftermath of disaster. J Trauma Stress 2004;17(5):363–72.

[8] Newman E, Kaloupek DG. The risks and benefits of participating in trauma-focused research studies. J Trauma Stress 2004;17(5):383–94.

[9] North CS, Pfefferbaum B. Research on the mental health effects of terrorism. JAMA 2002;288(5): 633–6.

[10] Rosenstein DL. Decision-making capacity and disaster research. J Trauma Stress 2004;17(5): 373–81.

[11] Levine C. The concept of vulnerability in disaster research. J Trauma Stress 2004;17(5):395–402.

[12] Kilpatrick DG. The ethics of disaster research: a special section. J Trauma Stress 2004;17(5):361–2.

[13] Fothergill A, Maestas EG, Darlington JD. Race, ethnicity and disasters in the United States: a review of the literature. Disasters 1999;23(2):156–73.

[14] Natural Hazards Center. University of Colorado, Boulder. Available at: http://www.colorado.edu/hazards/research/qr/guidelines.html. Accessed August 18, 2007.

[15] Disaster Research Education and Mentoring (DREM) Center. Available at: http://www.disasterresearch.org. Accessed August 18, 2007.

[16] Research Education in Disaster Mental Health (REDMH). Available at: http://www.redmh.org. Accessed August 18, 2007.

[17] National Child Traumatic Stress Network (NCTSN). Available at: http://www.nctsnet.org. Accessed August 18, 2007.

[18] Murphy F. Preparing for the field: developing competence as an ethnographic field worker. Nurse Res 2005;12(3):52–60.

[19] Borbasi S, Jackson D, Wilkes L. Fieldwork in nursing research: positionality, practicalities and predicaments. J Adv Nurs 2005;51(5):493–501.

[20] Safety guidelines for field researchers. Available at: http://www.ehs.berkeley.edu/pubs/fieldresearchsfty.pdf. Accessed August 18, 2007.

[21] Safety issues for field workers. Available at: http://www.aes.ucdavis.edu/Research/FieldSafety/workers.htm. Accessed August 18, 2007.

ELSEVIER
SAUNDERS

Crit Care Nurs Clin N Am 20 (2008) 121–131

CRITICAL CARE
NURSING CLINICS
OF NORTH AMERICA

# Military Nursing Research: Translation to Disaster Response and Day-to-Day Critical Care Nursing

Elizabeth J. Bridges, PhD, RN, CCNS, Lt Col, USAFR, NC[a,b,c,*],
Joseph Schmelz, PhD, RN, Lt Col, USAF, NC (Ret)[d],
Patricia Watts Kelley, PhD, RN, FNP, GNP, CAPT, NC, USN[e]

[a]Clinical Investigations Facility, 60th Medical Group, Travis AFB, CA, USA
[b]Biobehavioral Nursing and Health Systems, University of Washington School of Nursing,
Health Sciences Building, 1959 NE Pacific Street, Box 357266, Seattle, WA 98103, USA
[c]University of Washington Medical Center, 1959 NE Pacific Street, Box 357266, Seattle, WA 98103, USA
[d]School of Nursing, University of Texas Health Science Center at San Antonio (UTHSCSA),
Mail Code 7830, 7703 Floyd Curl Drive, San Antonio, TX 78229-3900, USA
[e]TriService Nursing Research Program, Uniformed Services University of the Health Sciences,
4301 Jones Bridge Road, Bethesda, MD 20814-4799, USA

A challenge facing health care providers called on to respond to disasters, humanitarian crises, or military operations (ie, contingencies) is, where to begin? How do you begin to identify areas where care will be the same or different and does any evidence support modifying practice in these potentially austere environments? Lessons learned from the military may be useful in answering this question [1–4]. This article presents a framework for identifying areas of critical care nursing practice that may be similar or different in a contingency setting. Using examples from disasters and military operations, three areas of patient care (cardiopulmonary resuscitation [CPR], hypothermia prevention, and invasive pressure monitoring), which are different in an austere contingency environment, are presented to demonstrate the use of this framework. Lessons learned from military nursing research related to these areas that can be translated into disaster response or day-to-day critical care are presented.

## Where to begin? Determining nursing care requirements during a contingency

Where to begin? To answer this question, a framework using a series of questions was created by a team of Air Force nurse researchers to identify topics for military-unique nursing research. The questions that were asked included:

1. What nursing care do we provide on a day-to-day basis that we will also provide in a deployed military, disaster, or humanitarian environment?
2. What are the characteristics of the patients cared for during different contingency operations?
3. What are the characteristics of the contingency environment?
4. How does the environment affect the care provided?

This work was supported by grants from the TriService Nursing Research Program (N00-019, N01-012, N02-P04). The views expressed in this article are those of the authors and do not reflect the official policy or position of the Department of the Air Force, the Department of the Navy, the TriService Nursing Research Program, the Department of Defense, or the United States Government.

* Corresponding author. Biobehavioral Nursing and Health Systems, University of Washington School of Nursing, Health Sciences Building, 1959 NE Pacific Street, Box 357266, Seattle, WA 98103.

E-mail address: ebridges@u.washington.edu (E.J. Bridges).

0899-5885/08/$ - see front matter. Published by Elsevier Inc.
doi:10.1016/j.ccell.2007.10.011

Although this framework was initially designed to identify military-unique research questions [4], the results of this work have direct application to disaster response and, in some cases, to day-to-day critical care nursing. Table 1 provides examples of the types of questions asked and the research questions designed to address these questions. This research, which was funded by the TriService Nursing Research Program (TSNRP), provides evidence to guide practice under the austere and unique conditions experienced in any contingency setting.

## Cardiopulmonary resuscitation

Much of the literature describing care provided immediately after a disaster, or during a humanitarian relief effort or military operation, focuses on individuals who suffer traumatic or psychologic injuries. However, individuals who are not directly affected by the disaster may also require care. For example, a unique group of patients who may present after a disaster are those with acute coronary syndrome or sudden cardiac arrest. The Great Hanshin-Awaji earthquake in Japan in 1995, which registered 7.2 on the Richter scale, affected 3.5 million people and caused 5480 deaths and 41,000 injuries, and left 342,000 homeless, with most of the casualties suffering injuries from falling debris and being crushed [8]. After the earthquake, there was also a three-fold increase in acute myocardial infarctions (AMIs) [9] and sudden cardiac arrest increased by 50% [11,12]. The increased rate of deaths may have been in part due to the loss of services. In the Kobe, Japan, region, 103 of the 112 hospitals (34,614 inpatient beds) [8] and 763 of the 1363 clinics were damaged. In 42 medical facilities affected by the earthquake, 886 patients required intensive care, and 40% of those patients had to be transferred to medical facilities outside the region [8].

The 1994 Northridge, California, earthquake killed 61 people, injured 7000, and left 51,000 homeless. Of the 79 coronary care units in the Los Angeles area, 7 were closed temporarily or completely because of damage, and 8 of 91 acute care hospitals (1670 inpatient beds) had to be evacuated within 24 hours of the earthquake. One hospital evacuated all its patients to an open parking lot [13]. On the day of the Northridge earthquake, admissions for AMI increased by 110%; deaths due to sudden cardiac arrest increased from an average of 4.6 per day to 24 on the day of the earthquake [14,15].

Hurricane Katrina struck the United States on 29 August 2005. This catastrophe resulted in the evacuation of more than 1 million individuals. From 1 to 22 September 2005, exacerbations of chronic medical problems, which included cardiovascular disease, accounted for 33% of all health care visits at the medical clinics in hurricane evacuation centers [16]. At an evacuation center in Austin, Texas, 50% of the adults had an acute condition on arrival and 59% reported living with a chronic condition [17], and at the Houston Astrodome, the primary chronic disease treated was uncontrolled hypertension [18].

Acts of terrorism can also increase the incidence of cardiac events [19,20]. Although cardiac death rates did not increase in the New York City area after the September 11 attacks [21], in the month after the attack, in 200 patients with implantable cardiac defibrillators who lived in the New York City area, the number of serious tachyarrhythmias suffered by these individuals increased 2.3 fold [22], and in 132 individuals with implantable cardiac defibrillators living in Florida, the incidence of defibrillator shocks increased 2.8 fold, with each individual suffering an average of 2.4 events (primarily ventricular tachycardia) [23].

The ability to respond to an increased number of patients presenting with AMIs and sudden cardiac arrests after a disaster may be complicated by the acute loss of medical facilities, which requires that care (including CPR) be provided in austere conditions where simple supplies such as backboards are not readily available. In military field hospitals and during military medical air transport, the first beds available are military stretchers (ie, North Atlantic Treaty Organization [NATO] field litter). In many emergency medical facilities, including those supported by the National Disaster Management System, the NATO litter is also used (Fig. 1). The NATO litter, which is a canvas stretcher that is 22 in wide and 72 in long (Fig. 2), has two additional straps of material (crossmembers) located 14 in from the head and foot of the litter that stabilize it. In previous research on the skin interface pressure on the NATO litter [24], it was noted that these two straps of material become very stiff when distended. The authors' research team wondered if this stiff material could act as a surrogate backboard for CPR. A study using an animal model was conducted to determine if CPR could be performed effectively on a NATO litter without a backboard, compared with CPR with

Table 1
Examples of use of a framework to identify areas of critical care nursing practice in contingency operations and translation from military to civilian health care

| What nursing care is provided on a day-to-day basis that will also be provided in a contingency operation? | What are the characteristics of the contingency environment? How does the environment affect the care provided? | Examples of research questions addressed to provide evidence-based recommendations for care under contingency conditions |
|---|---|---|
| Chest tube maintenance | Limited space on a litter for positioning drainage tube | What is the best position for chest tubes to facilitate fluid removal from the chest [5]? |
| Endotracheal suctioning | Decreased barometric pressure and oxygen at altitude | Do ground-based protocols to prevent suction-induced hypoxemia provide the same protection at altitude [6]? What is the optimal safe suction pressure at altitude [7]? |
| Prevention of pressure ulcers | Hospital bed replaced by military canvas stretcher | What is the most effective method to decrease the risk of pressure ulcer formation on a NATO litter [24]? |
| Invasive pressure monitoring | Decreased barometric pressure at altitude causes gas bubbles in pressure monitoring system to expand | What is the effect of altitude-induced gas bubble expansion on the dynamic response characteristics of invasive pressure monitoring systems [44]? Do you need to rezero a pressure monitoring system with ascent to altitude (or any change in barometric pressure) [44]? Does an altitude-sensitive algorithm for preparation of a pressure monitoring system improve the dynamic response characteristics of the system [44]? |
| Prevention of hypothermia | Temperature onboard military cargo aircraft decreases to 50°F to 60°F | Can you describe the thermal environmental characteristics onboard a military cargo aircraft used for aeromedical evacuation [10]? |
|  | Hypothermia prevention strategies must be lightweight, use minimal electricity, and not interfere with aircraft equipment | What hypothermia prevention strategies are most effective in preventing hypothermia in a trauma victim in a contingency environment [37,38]? |
| CPR | Evacuation of fixed medical facilities or care provided in a field hospital and onboard aircraft, which are austere environments | Can CPR be performed effectively on a NATO litter or decontamination litter with or without a backboard [25]? |
|  | Use of canvas stretchers (NATO litter) Lack of backboards | What is the effect on survival of a 2-minute delay to move a patient to the floor (hard surface) versus initiation of resuscitation on NATO litter without a backboard [25]? |

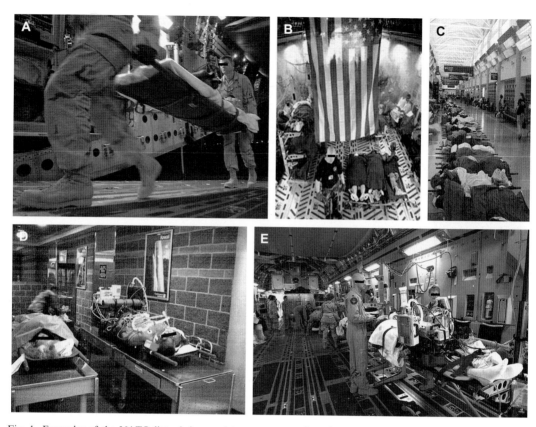

Fig. 1. Examples of the NATO litter being used to transport patients in military and disaster response operations. Clockwise from top left. (*A*) Casualty being brought onboard aircraft on NATO litter. (US Air Force photo/Staff Sgt. Michael R. Holzworth.) (*B*) Medical evacuees from Hurricane Katrina loaded on NATO litters on C-17 cargo aircraft. (US Air Force photo/Master Sgt. Lance Cheung.) (*C*) Medical evacuees awaiting transport at the New Orleans airport after Hurricane Katrina. (*D*) Critically ill evacuees being prepared for transport out of New Orleans by a USAF Critical Care Air Transport team. (*E*) Critically injured casualty onboard C-17 cargo aircraft. (US Air Force photo/Airman 1st Class Nathan Doza.)

a backboard on the litter or on a hard surface (simulating the floor) [25]. Additionally, the efficacy of CPR was studied on a special mesh litter used during decontamination, with and without a backboard.

The results indicated no significant difference in the efficacy of CPR on the NATO litter and decontamination litter with a backboard or on the NATO litter without the backboard if the crossmember was used as surrogate backboard. However, CPR efficacy was decreased on the decontamination litter without a backboard (Fig. 3). The most efficacious CPR was on the hard surface; however, the efficacy of CPR on the hard surface was significantly different only from the CPR performed on the decontamination litter without a backboard.

The next question that was asked was, What was the cost in terms of survival associated with a delay in CPR caused when moving the patient off the litter and to the floor? This research is important because the most recent CPR guidelines indicate that CPR must be initiated immediately [26]. It takes a minimum of 2 to 3 minutes to move a patient safely to the floor. For every 1 minute delay in the initiation of CPR, survival from a witnessed ventricular fibrillation arrest decreases by 7% to 10% [27]; thus, the delay in CPR to move a patient to the floor would potentially decrease survival by 14% to 30%. To simulate a typical response to a cardiac arrest, ventricular fibrillation was induced for 2 minutes, after which the animal subjects on the NATO litter (without a backboard) were defibrillated, and CPR was

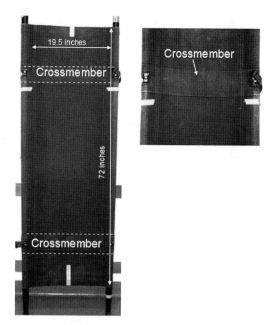

Fig. 2. The NATO litter, which is a canvas litter used in military, disaster, and humanitarian responses. The litter has two straps of material (crossmembers) that stiffen with distention (*inset*) and are useful as a surrogate CPR backboard.

initiated if defibrillation was not successful. To simulate moving a patient to the floor, an additional 2-minute delay in defibrillation and CPR was observed for the second group. The results of the study were consistent with other research that demonstrates increased mortality with a delay in CPR and defibrillation. The survival rate was 87% for the NATO litter group and only 47% for the delayed initiation group (hard surface group).

*Implications and recommendations for practice*

Based on this research, it appears that CPR and cardiac resuscitation can be performed on the NATO litter. If movement of the patient to the floor is necessary because of an inability to gain access to the patient due to the litter position, defibrillation should be attempted before moving the patient. If resuscitation is possible on the NATO litter and a backboard is not available, the patient should be repositioned so that his/her sternum is perpendicular to the crossmember. This repositioning will allow for maximum efficacy of chest compressions and puts the head and airway in a slightly extended position, which may facilitate ventilation.

### Hypothermia prevention in trauma victims

The initial care of trauma patients includes interventions to prevent or treat the deadly triad of trauma: hypothermia, coagulopathy, and acidosis. In trauma victims, hypothermia ($<35°C$) increases the risk for morbidity and mortality [28–30]. In addition, in trauma and surgical patients, hypothermia increases fluid volume requirements [31], causes coagulopathies [32,33], impairs wound

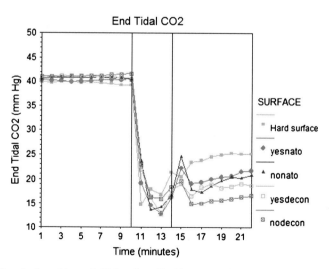

Fig. 3. Efficacy of CPR as indicated by end tidal carbon dioxide ($ETCO_2$) on various support surfaces (higher $ETCO_2$ indicates more efficacious CPR). Nonato, NATO litter without a backboard; nodecon, decontamination litter without a backboard; yesdecon, decontamination litter with a backboard; yesnato, NATO litter with a backboard.

healing and increases wound infections [34]. At a military field hospital in Southeast Asia, the incidence of hypothermia ($<36°C$) in trauma victims was 18% [35]. Anecdotal reports from Iraq and Afghanistan indicate that hypothermia can occur despite ambient temperatures that are 96°F on average and often exceed 120°F during the summer months. Casualties at the field hospital who were hypothermic on admission were more likely to be hypotensive, tachycardic, acidotic, and have a lower Glasgow Coma Scale score and hematocrit [35]. In addition, those who were hypothermic required more aggressive surgical management, had higher use of blood products, and experienced increased overall mortality [35,36].

In a hospital setting, hypothermia prevention is commonly performed using three methods: passive protection (eg, blankets or reflective blankets), active warming of the skin (eg, forced-air warmers or conductive warming blankets), and core body warming (eg, intravenous [IV] fluid warmers). However, in a contingency setting, the availability of blankets and electricity may be limited and weight restrictions preclude the transport of large quantities of these warming devices. In addition, if a patient is transported by air, an added challenge is that the warming device cannot interfere with the aircraft's electronic equipment. The authors' research team was challenged to identify effective hypothermia prevention techniques using equipment that was lightweight, mobile, required minimal electricity (ideally battery powered), and was safe to use onboard an aircraft (helicopter or plane).

A series of studies was conducted to evaluate various products that were advertised to prevent hypothermia under austere conditions [37,38]. The studies used a well-established animal model of hemorrhagic shock under environmental conditions consistent with long-distance military aeromedical transport (50°F with 0.2 m/sec airflow). To simulate severe trauma, the animals underwent a 50% hemorrhage to a mean arterial pressure of 30 mm Hg (class IV shock), then were resuscitated using an ambient temperature colloid (hetastarch 6%). After initial resuscitation, the animal was left uncovered (control group) or covered with a double-layer wool blanket or a baffled reflective blanket (Blizzard Blanket, Blizzard Protection Systems, Gwynned, United Kingdom). In the first study, the fluids were either administered at ambient temperature (Hetastarch at 50°F) with the blood administered at 4°C (simulating blood

being brought straight from the blood bank) or by way of the Thermal Angel (Estill Medical Technologies, Inc., Dallas, Texas). The Thermal Angel is a portable fluid warmer that heats fluids to between 81°F and 91°F [39]. In the second study, active warming was provided with the Chillbuster (Model 8100; Thermogear, Inc., Tigard, Oregon), which is an 8-pound portable electric/battery optional warming blanket. Fig. 4 reflects the changes in core body temperature using the various warming methods.

### Implications and recommendations for practice

The studies demonstrate that passive warming using wool blankets does not prevent hypothermia. Additionally, the use of a reflective blanket may decrease the severity of hypothermia, but does not prevent hypothermia. Active warming (eg, IV fluid warming or skin warming) used in combination with a passive method is effective in preventing hypothermia. Further research is ongoing using the Blizzard Blanket plus the Ready-Heat (TechTrade LLC, New York), which is a carbon-fiber blanket with an embedded chemical warming pack that is activated when exposed to oxygen. This blanket, which takes approximately 30 minutes to reach 104°F, in combination with the Blizzard Blanket, prevented hypothermia in a hemorrhagic shock model under extreme conditions consistent with open-door military helicopter transport (37°F with 8 m/sec wind speed). (Schmelz and DeJong, personal communication, 2007). Although these combined warming approaches are effective in preventing hypothermia, caution must be taken to avoid possible thermal injuries, and careful monitoring of the patient's temperature is needed to prevent hyperthermia, particularly in casualties with traumatic brain injury [40]. The results of these studies have already informed hypothermia-prevention strategies in use in current military operations.

### Invasive pressure monitoring

During long-distance aeromedical transport, the use of invasive pressure monitoring is essential because the ability to auscultate a blood pressure is nearly impossible because of the aircraft noise. Most critically injured casualties evacuated from current military operations in Iraq and Afghanistan are transported with an arterial line [41].

The standards for setting up and maintaining invasive pressure monitoring and the performance

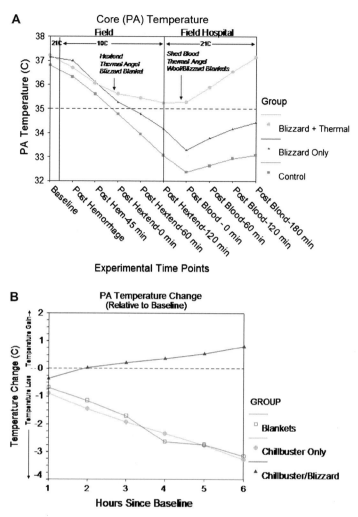

Fig. 4. (*A*) Efficacy of various warming methods (wool blankets, Blizzard Blanket, Thermal Angel) on the prevention of hypothermia in an animal hemorrhagic shock model. Ambient temperature was adjusted from 50°F (10°C) to 72°F (21°C) to simulate movement from the field to a military field hospital [37]. (*B*) Efficacy of wool blankets, Chillbuster, and Chillbuster plus Blizzard Blanket on the prevention of hypothermia in an animal hemorrhagic shock model. The experiment took place in a 50°F environment [38].

of invasive pressure monitoring are well established [42]. During preparation of invasive pressure monitoring lines, steps to remove all air bubbles are outlined, in addition to recommendations to simplify the system (eg, removal of excess tubing). These steps take on greater importance when preparing a pressure monitoring system for a patient who will be transported by air [43]. With ascent to altitude, barometric pressure decreases, causing gas bubbles to expand. For example, ascent from sea level to 8000 feet cabin altitude (a common cabin altitude for pressurized aircraft) causes a gas bubble to expand by 35%.

At sea level, air bubbles in the system causes the system to be underdamped (eg, systolic blood pressure overestimated and diastolic blood pressure underestimated) or unacceptable (blood pressure measurements cannot be used to guide practice). With ascent to altitude, gas bubble expansion further worsens the dynamic response characteristics of the system. Regardless of the location of care (eg, onboard a cargo aircraft or in a fixed medical facility), steps need to be taken to ensure that all air bubbles are removed from the pressure monitoring system. In addition, more complex pressure systems, such as systems with a blood reservoir, have worse dynamic response characteristics compared with a straight pressure line, with the reservoir systems generally underdamped [42,44,45].

A technique known as a "rocket flush" eliminates air bubbles from the pressure monitoring system [46] before the system is connected to the patient. A rocket flush is performed by drawing up 10 mL of sterile solution and, after initial preparation of the pressure monitoring system, the system is vigorously flushed with the solution, which is introduced through the proximal stopcock (next to the transducer). The effectiveness of the rocket flush was evaluated in pressure monitoring systems with a VAMP device (Edwards Lifesciences, Irvine, California) at sea level and with ascent to altitude [44]. The pressure systems were prepared using current recommendations, and the dynamic response characteristics of the system were evaluated before and after the rocket flush. As demonstrated in Fig. 5, using the standard protocol, 41% of the pressure systems were underdamped and 59% were adequate. After a single rocket flush, 8% of the systems were underdamped, 88% were adequate, and 4% were optimal.

*Implications and recommendations for practice*

Based on these results, the current protocol for the set-up of invasive pressure monitoring systems was modified to emphasize steps during set-up to eliminate air bubbles from the system (Box 1). Of great importance, because of the risk for retrograde air embolization, the rocket flush should never be performed if the pressure monitoring system is attached to a patient.

### TriService Nursing Research Program

The research presented in this article was primarily funded by grants from the TSNRP. TSNRP supports military nursing research and evidence-based practice, and competitive funding is available to active duty, Reserve and Guard personnel, and retired military nurses who are doctorally prepared. This article demonstrates how important TSNRP's support is in studying topics that initially appear to have sole relevance to the military, because the results of this military research may be translated into disaster response and civilian health care practice.

### Summary

Lessons from military health care practice and research can be translated to civilian disaster response and day-to-day civilian health care delivery. This article presented a framework that is useful in identifying care requirements in response to military, disaster, and humanitarian contingencies. This article also demonstrated that health care is needed not only for those directly affected

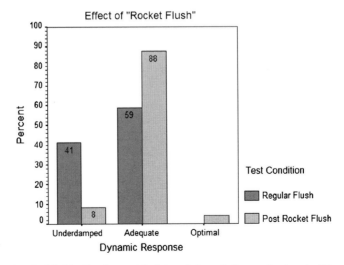

Fig. 5. Effect of a "rocket flush" (10 mL saline rapidly injected through the proximal port of the pressure system to remove microbubbles) on the dynamic response characteristics of an invasive pressure monitoring system. The systems prepared using the rocket flush provided reliable pressure measurements 92% of the time, in contrast to only 59% with the standard pressure line preparation.

**Box 1. Protocol for practice: preparation of invasive pressure monitoring system**

1. Wash hands.
2. Gather supplies (normal saline IV bag, pressure monitoring kit, 10-mL luer lock syringe, pressure bag with self-venting gauge).
3. Prime pressure monitoring system to remove all air.
   a. Remove pressure monitoring kit from package, open blood salvage reservoir, tighten connections, close roller clamp, turn stopcock OFF to patient (off toward distal end), and remove vented (white) stopcock cap.
   b. Remove IV port cover and pressure monitoring line spike cover.
   c. Invert IV bag to orient bag upside down and, using sterile technique, insert spike into IV bag.
   d. Leave the spiked bag upside down, open roller clamp and simultaneously pull (activate) fast-flush device (pigtail) continuously while gently squeezing to apply pressure to IV bag to clear air slowly from IV bag and drip chamber. Completely fill the drip chamber with IV fluid.
   e. Turn IV bag upright once fluid is advanced sufficiently past the drip chamber.
   f. Apply gentle pressure to the IV bag (or hang the bag ~30 in above distal end of tubing) and pull fast-flush device; advance fluid, priming the stopcock.
   g. Orient fluid so that air will be completely removed by the advancing fluid (ie, tilt distal end of reservoir upright at 45° angle).
   h. Pull (activate) fast-flush device while holding blood reservoir at angle, continuing to flush until the entire line is primed.
   i. Close blood reservoir, advancing all reservoir fluid through line.
   j. Perform rocket flush. (DO NOT PERFORM ROCKET FLUSH IF PRESSURE LINE IS ATTACHED TO PATIENT.)
      1. Turn stopcock off to distal end of catheter ("off to patient").
      2. Attach a 10-mL syringe to the stopcock near the transducer using sterile technique and slowly withdraw IV fluid to fill syringe.
      3. Turn stopcock off to transducer ("off to monitor").
      4. Flush line quickly with 10 mL normal saline from syringe to remove any remaining air bubbles; avoid instilling any air into the line.
      5. Turn stopcock off to port and remove syringe.
      6. Cap stopcock using sterile technique with solid blue cap.
4. Place IV bag into self-venting pressure bag and inflate to reach 250 to 300 mm Hg and recheck for air in line.
5. Inspect line, remove any remaining air by flushing line using rocket flush, as indicated by the dynamic response of the system (goal: Adequate or Optimal system) [42].

---

*Data from* Bridges E, Evers KG, Schmelz JO, et al. Invasive pressure monitoring at altitude. Crit Care Med 2005;22:A13.

by a disaster (eg, trauma from collapsed building) but also for those who are indirectly affected (eg, increased incidence of sudden cardiac arrests and AMI).

### References

[1] Grissom TE, Farmer JC. The provision of sophisticated critical care beyond the hospital: lessons from physiology and military experiences that apply to civil disaster medical response. Crit Care Med 2005;33:S13–21.
[2] Farmer JC, Carlton PK Jr. Providing critical care during a disaster: the interface between disaster response agencies and hospitals. Crit Care Med 2006;34:S56–9.

[3] Sariego J. CCATT: a military model for civilian disaster management. Disaster Manag Response 2006;4:114–7.

[4] Schmelz JO, Bridges EJ, Duong DN, et al. Care of the critically ill patient in a military unique environment: a program of research. Crit Care Nurs Clin North Am 2003;15:171–81.

[5] Schmelz JO, Johnson D, Norton JM, et al. Effects of position of chest drainage tube on volume drained and pressure. Am J Crit Care 1999;8:319–23.

[6] Schmelz J, Stone K, Johnson AD, et al. Preventing suctioning induced hypoxemia at altitude. Am J Crit Care 2000;9:218.

[7] Bridges E, Schmelz J, Stone K, et al. Endotracheal suctioning at altitude: implications for practice. Am J Crit Care 2000;9:218.

[8] Tanaka H, Iwai A, Oda J, et al. Overview of evacuation and transport of patients following the 1995 Hanshin-Awaji earthquake. J Emerg Med 1998;16: 439–44.

[9] Kario K, McEwen BS, Pickering TG. Disasters and the heart: a review of the effects of earthquake-induced stress on cardiovascular disease. Hypertens Res 2003;26:355–67.

[10] Bridges E. Thermal stress and the human response to thermal stress with litter position on the C-141 Starlifter and C-17 Globemaster II. Bethesda, MD: Tri-Service Nursing Research Program. 2005.

[11] Kario K, Ohashi T. Increased coronary heart disease mortality after the Hanshin-Awaji earthquake among the older community on Awaji Island. Tsuna Medical Association. J Am Geriatr Soc 1997;45: 610–3.

[12] Ogawa K, Tsuji I, Shiono K, et al. Increased acute myocardial infarction mortality following the 1995 Great Hanshin-Awaji earthquake in Japan. Int J Epidemiol 2000;29:449–55.

[13] Schultz CH, Koenig KL, Lewis RJ. Implications of hospital evacuation after the Northridge, California, earthquake. N Engl J Med 2003;348:1349–55.

[14] Leor J, Poole WK, Kloner RA. Sudden cardiac death triggered by an earthquake. N Engl J Med 1996;334:413–9.

[15] Kloner RA, Leor J, Poole WK, et al. Population-based analysis of the effect of the Northridge Earthquake on cardiac death in Los Angeles County, California. J Am Coll Cardiol 1997;30:1174–80.

[16] Morbidity surveillance after Hurricane Katrina – Arkansas, Louisiana, Mississippi, and Texas, September 2005. MMWR Morb Mortal Wkly Rep 2006;55:727–31.

[17] Vest JR, Valadez AM. Health conditions and risk factors of sheltered persons displaced by Hurricane Katrina. Prehospital Disaster Med 2006;21:55–8.

[18] Gavagan TF, Smart K, Palacio H, et al. Hurricane Katrina: medical response at the Houston Astrodome/Reliant Center Complex. South Med J 2006; 99:933–9.

[19] Qureshi EA, Merla V, Steinberg J, et al. Terrorism and the heart: implications for arrhythmogenesis and coronary artery disease. Card Electrophysiol Rev 2003;7:80–4.

[20] Bhattacharyya MR, Steptoe A. Emotional triggers of acute coronary syndromes: strength of evidence, biological processes, and clinical implications. Prog Cardiovasc Dis 2007;49:353–65.

[21] Chi JS, Poole WK, Kandefer SC, et al. Cardiovascular mortality in New York City after September 11, 2001. Am J Cardiol 2003;92:857–61.

[22] Steinberg JS, Arshad A, Kowalski M, et al. Increased incidence of life-threatening ventricular arrhythmias in implantable defibrillator patients after the World Trade Center attack. J Am Coll Cardiol 2004;44:1261–4.

[23] Shedd OL, Sears SF Jr, Harvill JL, et al. The World Trade Center attack: increased frequency of defibrillator shocks for ventricular arrhythmias in patients living remotely from New York City. J Am Coll Cardiol 2004;44:1265–7.

[24] Bridges EJ, Schmelz JO, Mazer S. Skin interface pressure on the NATO litter. Mil Med 2003;168:280–6.

[25] Bridges E, Schmelz J, Woods S, et al. Efficacy of CPR on the NATO and decontamination litter with and without a backboard. Am J Crit Care 2004;13:257.

[26] 2005 International Consensus on Cardiopulmonary Resuscitation and Emergency Cardiovascular Care Science with Treatment Recommendations. Part 2: adult basic life support. Resuscitation 2005;67: 187–201.

[27] Larsen MP, Eisenberg MS, Cummins RO, et al. Predicting survival from out-of-hospital cardiac arrest: a graphic model. Ann Emerg Med 1993;22: 1652–8.

[28] Shafi S, Elliott AC, Gentilello L. Is hypothermia simply a marker of shock and injury severity or an independent risk factor for mortality in trauma patients? Analysis of a large national trauma registry. J Trauma 2005;59:1081–5.

[29] Martin RS, Kilgo PD, Miller PR, et al. Injury-associated hypothermia: an analysis of the 2004 National Trauma Data Bank. Shock 2005;24:114–8.

[30] Wang HE, Callaway CW, Peitzman AB, et al. Admission hypothermia and outcome after major trauma. Crit Care Med 2005;33:1296–301.

[31] Gentilello LM, Jurkovich GJ, Stark MS, et al. Is hypothermia in the victim of major trauma protective or harmful? A randomized, prospective study. Ann Surg 1997;226:439–47.

[32] Krause KR, Howells GA, Buhs CL, et al. Hypothermia-induced coagulopathy during hemorrhagic shock. Am Surg 2000;66:348–54.

[33] Watts DD, Trask A, Soeken K, et al. Hypothermic coagulopathy in trauma: effect of varying levels of hypothermia on enzyme speed, platelet function, and fibrinolytic activity. J Trauma 1998;44:846–54.

[34] Dellinger EP. Roles of temperature and oxygenation in prevention of surgical site infection. Surg Infect (Larchmt) 2006;7(Suppl 3):s27–32.

[35] Arthurs Z, Cuadrado D, Beekley A, et al. The impact of hypothermia on trauma care at the 31st combat support hospital. Am J Surg 2006;191:610–4.

[36] Eastridge BJ, Owsley J, Sebesta J, et al. Admission physiology criteria after injury on the battlefield predict medical resource utilization and patient mortality. J Trauma 2006;61:820–3.

[37] Bridges E, Schmelz J, Evers K. Efficacy of the Blizzard Blanket or Blizzard Blanket plus Thermal Angel in preventing hypothermia in a hemorrhagic shock victim (Sus scrofa) under operational conditions. Mil Med 2007;172:17–23.

[38] Schmelz JO, Bridges EJ, Wallace CM, et al. Comparison of three strategies for preventing hypothermia in critically injured casualties during aeromedical evacuation. Mil Med 2007;172:322–6.

[39] Dubick MA, Brooks DE, Macaitis JM, et al. Evaluation of commercially available fluid-warming devices for use in forward surgical and combat areas. Mil Med 2005;170:76–82.

[40] The Brain Trauma Foundation. The American Association of Neurological Surgeons. The Joint Section on Neurotrauma and Critical Care. Critical pathway for the treatment of established intracranial hypertension. J Neurotrauma 2000;17:537–8.

[41] Bridges E, Evers K. Preliminary report: critical care air transport–Operation Iraqi Freedom (Oct 2001–Jun 2004). Bethesda, MD: TriService Nursing Research Program. 2005.

[42] Bridges E, Middleton R. Direct arterial vs oscillometric monitoring of blood pressure: stop comparing and pick one (a decision-making algorithm). Crit Care Nurse 1997;17:58–72.

[43] Pierce PF, Evers KG. Global presence: USAF aeromedical evacuation and critical care air transport. Crit Care Nurs Clin North Am 2003;15:221–31.

[44] Bridges E, Evers KG, Schmelz J, et al. Invasive pressure monitoring at altitude. Crit Care Med 2005;33:A13.

[45] Gore S, Middleton R, Bridges E. Analysis of an algorithm to guide decision making regarding direct and oscillometric blood pressure measurement. Am J Respir Crit Care Med 1995;151:A331.

[46] Promonet C, Anglade D, Menaouar A, et al. Time-dependent pressure distortion in a catheter-transducer system: correction by fast flush. Anesthesiology 2000;92:208–18.

ELSEVIER
SAUNDERS

Crit Care Nurs Clin N Am 20 (2008) 133–137

CRITICAL CARE
NURSING CLINICS
OF NORTH AMERICA

# Index

*Note:* Page numbers of article titles are in **boldface** type.

# Moving?

## Make sure your subscription moves with you!

To notify us of your new address, find your **Clinics Account Number** (located on your mailing label above your name), and contact customer service at:

E-mail: elspcs@elsevier.com

800-654-2452 (subscribers in the U.S. & Canada)
407-345-4000 (subscribers outside of the U.S. & Canada)

Fax number: 407-363-9661

**Elsevier Periodicals Customer Service**
6277 Sea Harbor Drive
Orlando, FL  32887-4800

*To ensure uninterrupted delivery of your subscription, please notify us at least 4 weeks in advance of move.

ELSEVIER